DEPARTMENT OF HEALTH

On the State of
THE PUBLIC HEALTH

THE ANNUAL REPORT OF
THE CHIEF MEDICAL OFFICER OF
THE DEPARTMENT OF HEALTH
FOR THE YEAR 1992

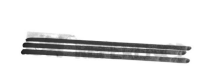

LONDON
HMSO

CONTENTS

iv

INTRODUCTION

Rt Hon Virginia Bottomley MP
Secretary of State for Health

Madam,

I have pleasure in submitting my Report on the State of the Public Health for 1992, together with some comments on the more important developments and events in the first half of 1993. This Report is the 135th of the series which began in 1858.

There were considerable improvements in health over the year: the perinatal and infant mortality rates were the lowest ever recorded and immunisation uptake rates among children were the highest ever achieved. 1992 witnessed the publication, in July, of the White Paper *The Health of the Nation: a strategy for health in England*[1], a landmark for the improvement of health in this country. Much of this Report is taken up with activities relating to implementation of the strategy for health and future Reports will record the changes in health which occur and monitor the outcome of actions taken as part of this historic initiative. However, as I pointed out last year, the Report is not simply a document of record; it must also try to interpret changes in relation to factors which influence and determine health, and attempt to identify health matters where further improvements might be made. The Report must also draw attention to issues where action is required and to problems which have been identified. The format of the main Report has been altered slightly to meet these needs and to reflect the importance of the strategy for health. The importance attached to effective communication in public health matters is shown in this year's Report by the inclusion of contributions from three Regional Directors of Public Health.

The format of this introduction has been extensively revised so that it provides a summary to the whole Report. It first sets out long-term strategic aims; these are followed by a brief discussion of key developments in 1992 and early 1993; a progress report on action points highlighted in the 1991 Report; a note of new issues identified during 1992, which will be reviewed in future years; and, finally, an executive summary of the Report as a whole.

I wish to acknowledge the help and support given to me by numerous colleagues in the Department of Health and the Office of Population Censuses and Surveys in the preparation of this Report, and the assistance of Her Majesty's Stationery Office, Norwich, which arranged the printing and publication.

I am, Madam,
Your obedient servant

Kenneth C Calman
September 1993

LONG-TERM STRATEGIC AIMS

A clear statement of long-term aims is essential in developing a strategy to improve health, health care and quality of life. I have identified six issues as crucial to the nation's health, and they are consistent with current Government policy.

- *To promote efforts to ensure health for all*: All sections of the community should be able to achieve the best in health and health care. Identification of those factors that influence health and health care is central to this aim.

- *To achieve the targets in the strategy for health*: Most of the targets in the *Health of the Nation* White Paper[1] are long-term objectives, but it should be possible to identify short-term indicators of progress in all five key areas (coronary heart disease [CHD] and stroke, cancers, mental health, HIV/AIDS and sexual health, and accidents).

- *To involve patients and the public in choices and decision-making*: Empowerment of patients and the public is essential if ownership of change is to be achieved and an effective service delivered. The *Patient's Charter*[2] is part of this aim.

- *To establish an effective intelligence and information system for public health and clinical practice*: Such a system is essential to monitor, and to ensure an appropriate response to, public health problems and to identify changes in clinical practice which would be for the benefit of the community. The Public Health Network (see page 49) will have a key role.

- *To ensure a health service based on an assessment of health needs, quality of care, and effectiveness of outcome*: The Clinical Outcomes Group (see page 110) will be a central part of such assessments, which must include economic and resource issues.

- *To provide a highly professional team of staff*: Health care professionals and managers are the key to changing health and health care. A strong educational and research base must also be associated with clear values and high ethical standards.

HEALTH IN ENGLAND IN 1992

1992 saw the perinatal mortality rate at an all time low of 7.9 per 1,000 total births; the lowest ever recorded infant mortality rate of 6.5 per 1,000 live births (due to a considerable extent to the successful campaign on the sleeping position of infants); life expectancy continuing to increase; the highest ever immunisation rates and introduction of the *Haemophilus influenzae* type b (Hib) vaccine; advice on increased folate or folic acid intakes for women intending to become pregnant, to reduce the risk of neural tube defects; and several encouraging advances in the management of various diseases. However, improvements are not uniform and some black spots remain: suicides among young males have increased markedly in recent years; cigarette smoking continues to cause many health problems and smoking prevalence, particularly among young people, is not falling quickly enough; too many people drink excessive amounts of alcohol; diet and physical activity could be improved for most people; and notifications of drug addicts to the Home Office are at an all-time high.

Trends in health can also usefully be assessed from a longer term perspective. Between 1982 and 1992 the overall mortality rate fell by 17%, the fall being over 20% in those aged under 65 years. This reduction in mortality was associated with a marked increase in average life expectancy at birth from 71.3 years in 1982 to an estimated 73.8 years in 1992 in males, and from 77.2 years in 1982 to an estimated 79.2 years in 1992 in females. There have been striking falls in the death rates for certain major causes of death such as CHD and stroke, where the rates in people aged under 65 years fell by more than 30% between 1982 and 1992, and lung cancer in men, where death rates fell by more than 20% in the same period. Major improvements have also occurred over this period in rates of perinatal mortality (down by 32%) and infant mortality, which fell by 40%.

Against this background of improvement over the last decade, areas of particular concern remain - such as the absence of a decline in breast and lung cancer mortality rates in women, and the absence of a decline in the overall mortality rate in young adult males (to which deaths from AIDS and suicide have been major contributors). Variations in health in groups categorised by occupation, social class and ethnicity persist: for example, recent figures for infant mortality - based on OPCS information which links infant death records with information from the corresponding birth records - indicate rates (for births within marriage) about 80% higher in the lowest social class compared with the highest. Mortality data can only provide a limited although important view of health trends. The General Household Survey (GHS) provides some relevant information on trends in self-reported 'long-standing illness, disability and infirmity'. Levels reported in 1991 are little different from those reported 10 years earlier but substantially higher than rates reported 20 years ago. Changing expectations and perceptions may explain some of this change.

KEY ISSUES IN THIS REPORT

The strategy for health

1992 saw considerable activity to disseminate the messages of the *Health of the Nation* White Paper[1]. Implementation of the strategy and its monitoring will be undertaken by three committees; the Wider Health Working Group chaired by Baroness Cumberlege, Parliamentary Under Secretary of State for Health in the House of Lords; my Health of the Nation Working Group, which will consider the progress towards targets and identify new key areas; and the Chief Executive's Working Group on National Health Service (NHS) implementation of the strategy. There is also a Committee to co-ordinate the strategy across 11 Government Departments. The Health of the Nation initiative continued into 1993 with the publication of five key area handbooks[3,4,5,6,7] to outline activities that could be taken forward by NHS managers, and others, to achieve targets. A series of conferences in each of the English health Regions showed how much work was going on in constructing 'healthy alliances' and 'healthy settings'. In June 1993, priorities and planning guidance for the NHS[8] identified the importance to Regions of setting local targets and taking forward work to achieve these targets; this guidance was supported by the issue of a consultative document on local target setting in July 1993[9]. The first anniversary of the launch of the initiative was marked by a series of events including my challenge to the nation to take several steps towards better health, publication of handbooks on 'healthy alliances'[10] and ethnic health issues[11], and release of the results of the first English Health Survey[12].

Immunisation

Immunisation against *Haemophilus influenzae* type b (Hib) infections started in October 1992. Laboratory reports of meningitis and bacteraemia in children under the age of 12 months have fallen by 70% in the first quarter of 1993 compared with the same period in each of the last 3 years. Early assessments of immunisation coverage suggest that the acceptance of Hib vaccine has been remarkably good, and market research shows very high levels of awareness of Hib vaccine among mothers of young children.

HIV infection and AIDS

Prevention and surveillance of HIV infection remained public health priorities throughout 1992, as evidenced by the choice of HIV/AIDS and sexual health as a key area in the strategy for health[1]. The handbook on how to address the specific objectives and targets in this area was published in January 1993[6]. In the first half of 1993, the Department also issued revised guidance on the management of HIV-infected health care workers[13] and the UK Health Departments issued guidance on notifying patients of HIV-infected health care workers[14]. In June 1993, understanding of the epidemic was enhanced by the publication of new projections for the development of the epidemic up to 1997[15], which are in line with previous predictions. The projections, which will be discussed in more detail in next year's Report, give no cause for complacency.

PROGRESS ON ACTION POINTS IN THE 1991 REPORT

In last year's Report a number of issues were identified as needing further consideration. I will continue to draw attention to these issues in future years.

Health of black and ethnic minority groups

The special chapter on the health of black and ethnic minority groups has been taken forward in various ways - including conferences, workshops, new research, and the setting up of an Ethnic Health Task Force chaired by Baroness Cumberlege. Ethnic minority issues now have a firm base in the health service and beyond, and must continue to be given a high priority.

Communicable diseases

A long-standing fall in the incidence of tuberculosis had ceased and in some areas the number of notifications had begun to rise; the number of notifications increased during 1992 by a further 5%. A special programme of surveillance was instituted to allow decisions to be made about future policy. It was also noted that the number of *Shigella sonnei* infections, which cause diarrhoea and are usually spread by poor hygiene, had risen. Again, increased surveillance was initiated and, although the increase noted in the latter part of 1991 continued into 1992, the number of infections has since declined. A possible relation between gastrointestinal infections and water disconnections has been raised; there is no evidence at this stage that the two are connected, but further studies are in progress.

Clinical audit and outcomes of health care

During 1992 there was considerable activity in the Department of Health, health Regions and Districts and educational bodies, and by individual clinicians. There is a perceptible move towards clinical, as opposed to medical, audit and the benefits are already being seen in clinical practice. Continued progress, in conjunction with increased emphasis on the related issues of effectiveness and technology assessment, should be translated into better health care. To improve the effectiveness of health care, the Clinical Outcomes Group, chaired jointly by the Chief Nursing Officer and myself, has been set up to co-ordinate work on clinical audit and quality issues in clinical practice. It is multidisciplinary and closely linked with other effectiveness and quality initiatives. There will be two patient representatives on the group, and over the next year patient involvement in Regional and District audit committees will be monitored and the multidisciplinary nature of the audit process will be emphasised.

Medical education and manpower

A number of initiatives were started in the past year and will be developed further. The draft report of the Working Group on Specialist Medical Training[16] was issued for consultation in April 1993; its recommendations (if accepted) will have important implications for the training of medical staff and the way in which qualified medical staff work. Appropriate links with European medical training are essential and will be pursued. Further reductions in junior doctors' hours have been made, with only 245 junior doctors and dentists in England contracted to work more than 83 hours a week on 27 April 1993 - a fall of over 13,000, or 98%, since September 1990.

NEW ISSUES IDENTIFIED DURING 1992

Each year a small number of specific issues will be identified as topics to be returned to in future Reports. This year four topics have been identified.

Health of men

The special topic in this year's Report is the health of men, who continue to have a lower life expectancy than women. Although some diseases, such as prostatism, are obviously unique to men, the main differences in mortality and morbidity relate to variations in exposure to risk factors. Thus, there should be great potential for improvement in health in many areas, for example CHD and accidents. Further work is particularly needed on targeting health messages to men. Women seem to be more aware of their own bodies and pay more attention to health messages. Health messages for men may be more effectively transmitted through mothers or sisters, wives or girlfriends, but men must now be brought up to be more aware of their own bodies and not to be reluctant to seek help. The concept of 'healthy settings' in the strategy for health should improve workplace safety. It is to be hoped that Regions and Districts will investigate ways to promote the health of men over the next few years.

Cigarette smoking among children

This remains too high. Interesting work to prevent uptake and to assist young people to stop smoking was identified during the *Health of the Nation* conferences and will be taken forward.

Mentally disordered offenders

Since 1987, these Reports have emphasised the importance of continuity of care for people with serious mental illness when they leave hospital, not least to prevent a decline into dereliction, homelessness and crime[17,18,19]; they have also recorded developments to improve such care[20]. My Report for last year included mention of the initial findings of the Department of Health/Home Office review of services for mentally disordered offenders[21]. The completed findings of this important review (see page 122), and other research[22], emphasise the challenges that must be met to ensure that people with serious mental illness cannot fall through the net of care, and highlight the need to provide a range of services to meet the varied, and often considerable, health and social care requirements of those mentally disordered people who do offend.

Verocytotoxin-producing *Escherichia coli*

Over the last 10 years the incidence of disease due to verocytotoxin-producing *Escherichia coli* (VTEC), mainly serotype 0157, has been increasing in England and Wales. Children and elderly people are particularly susceptible and infection may result in acute renal failure in children. The main sources of the organism are not fully established and the Advisory Committee on the Microbiological Safety of Food is assessing the significance of VTEC as a foodborne pathogen and the need for any controls to reduce human illness.

EXECUTIVE SUMMARY

VITAL STATISTICS

Population size

The resident population of England at 30 June 1992 was 48.2 million, an increase of 0.3% compared with 1991.

Age and sex structure of the resident population

The populations at pre-school and school ages are now fairly stable. The population at younger working ages (16-44 years) has begun to decline, while that at older working ages is beginning to rise. The rapid increase in the number of people aged 85 years and over continues.

Fertility statistics - aspects of relevance for health care

In 1991, based on provisional data, an estimated 809,111 conceptions occurred to women resident in England. The overall conception rate reached 78.1 per 1,000 women aged 15-44 years in 1991. The conception rate among the under 16s decreased from 10.1 per 1,000 girls aged 13-15 years in 1990, to 9.3 in 1991. There were 651,784 live births in England in 1992, 1% less than in 1991. In 1992 births outside marriage accounted for 31% of all live births.

Mortality

There were 522,656 deaths registered in England in 1992, 2.1% fewer than in 1991. The crude mortality rate decreased from 11.1 per 1,000 population in 1991, to 10.8 in 1992.

Mortality rates for males aged 15-44 years increased by 8% between 1985 and 1990. Since 1990 this rate has decreased by 4%. Mortality rates among children have fallen dramatically since 1988.

In 1992 there were 5,541 suicides and undetermined deaths in England, the same level as in 1982. However, this apparent stability masks the fact that over this period male deaths have been increasing, whilst female deaths have been decreasing.

Infant and perinatal mortality

In 1992 in England, 4,259 babies died before the age of one year. The infant mortality rate was 6.5 per 1,000 live births, the lowest ever recorded. This fall was due to a 25% decrease in the post-neonatal mortality rate. 2,975 stillbirths were recorded in 1992, 198 of them because of a change in the legal definition of stillbirth, which came into force on 1 October. The perinatal mortality rate fell to its lowest level, at 7.9 per 1,000 total births (or 7.6 if the 198 stillbirths registered because of the change in legal definition are excluded).

Acute and chronic sickness

In 1991, 31% of respondents to the GHS reported a long-standing illness, 18% a limiting long-standing illness and 12% restricted activity in the two weeks before interview. The prevalence of reported long-standing illness increased during the 1980s. Towards the end of the decade the increase slowed, and then a slight fall occurred.

Trends in cancer incidence and mortality

For all cancers combined there was no change in incidence over the period 1978-88. However, lung cancer registration decreased among males but increased for females over this period. Overall cancer mortality has shown no decline in recent years but there has been a fall in the mortality rate for cancer of the stomach for both sexes.

Trends in reporting congenital malformations

According to provisional data for 1992, the rate for malformed live births in England decreased by 12% between 1991 and 1992, from 98.1 per 10,000 live births to 86.2. Over the same period, the rate for malformed stillbirths fell by 4%, from 2.8 per 10,000 total births to 2.7.

THE NATION'S HEALTH

Public health in England

The Department of Health (DH) continued to monitor closely the public health function during 1992. A national Public Health Network was set up to facilitate communication and to make more effective use of sources of public health expertise. In view of the changes resulting from the National Health Service and Community Care Act 1990[23], a small working group was established "to review HC(88)64 in the light of the NHS reforms and to develop new guidance by spring 1993". A series of meetings and seminars, attended by a wide variety of health professionals, were held to assist with policy development for future legislation on infectious disease control. Additional funding was provided for the training of doctors in the specialty of public health medicine and for continuing education for consultants in communicable disease control.

Smoking and health

Smoking is the single most important cause of preventable disease and premature death in England. The strategy for health[1] sets challenging targets for the reduction in smoking levels by the year 2000; if these are to be achieved, continued vigorous action is needed on several fronts. Adult smoking rates continue to fall, in prevalence and consumption, but the high risks of smoking and the wide range of diseases caused by smoking are still not fully appreciated by the public. Rates of smoking among children are not falling quickly enough, and the teenage anti-smoking programme is being widened to include families and to persuade parents who smoke that they should set a better example. The price of tobacco products also has a major impact on smoking, particularly among young people: tobacco taxes will be maintained at least in line with inflation.

There has been increasing awareness of harm from passive smoking. The strategy for health also includes specific objectives for the introduction of no-smoking policies in public places and workplaces, and steps have been taken to ensure that all National Health Service (NHS) premises are smoke-free apart from a limited number of separate smoking rooms.

Alcohol misuse

Alcohol consumption in sensible quantities and appropriate circumstances is not harmful, but excessive and inappropriate drinking beyond recommended safe limits contributes to a wide range of health and social problems. As national patterns of drinking change there is evidence of increasing public awareness about safe levels of drinking and the use of alcohol units. The strategy for health targets[1] to reduce the proportion of heavy drinkers spearhead a range of Government initiatives to deal with this problem.

Drug misuse

The total number of opioid addicts notified to the Home Office during 1992 was 24,700, the highest number yet recorded, continuing an upwards trend. However the proportion of addicts injecting drugs fell for the third year running, probably reflecting an increase in oral methadone prescribing. The impact of needle-syringe exchange schemes and health promotion about AIDS and drug misuse is reflected in continuing low HIV-seroprevalence figures among drug misusers. The strategy for health targets[1] emphasise a need for further reductions in needle sharing. Wider health promotion issues were successfully addressed in the European Drugs Prevention Week.

'Look After Your Heart' Programme
The 'Look After Your Heart' (LAYH) programme continues to be a focus for coronary heart disease (CHD) preventive activity in England through its national and local activities, which include the Workplace programme, the 'Enjoy healthy eating' campaign, LAYH Heartbeat Awards and 'LAYH Take Part' for physical activity.

Physical activity

The activity and fitness of English adults was assessed in the Allied Dunbar National Fitness Survey[24]. Seventy per cent of men and 80% of women do not achieve the levels of regular physical activity likely to provide a health benefit at their age, whereas 80% of men and women of all ages believed themselves to be physically fit and thought that they did do enough exercise to keep fit. Strategies to encourage appropriate levels of physical activity will be set up as part of the strategy for health initiative.

Nutrition

As part of the strategy for health, a Nutrition Task Force, comprising members from a wide range of industrial, academic and voluntary sectors, was set up to develop a plan of action to achieve the nutritional components to the key area targets for CHD and stroke[1]. The Committee on Medical Aspects of Food Policy published a Report on the nutrition of elderly people[25], which reviewed available information and made recommendations. Another Expert Group recommended increased folate or folic acid intakes for all women who wanted to become pregnant, to reduce the incidence of neural tube defects[26]. The report of the quinquennial national survey of infant feeding[27], commissioned by DH, was published by the Office of Population Censuses and Surveys (OPCS).

THE STRATEGY FOR HEALTH

The Health of the Nation White Paper

The White Paper *The Health of the Nation: a Strategy for Health in England*[1] was published in July 1992. It identified five key areas for priority action - CHD and stroke, cancers, mental illness, HIV/AIDS and sexual health, and accidents. These were selected after wide consultation following publication of the Green Paper *The Health of the Nation: a Consultative Document for Health in England* in 1991[28]. The White Paper sets out national objectives and sets 27 specific targets over five key areas and indicates the action which is needed to achieve the targets.

Key areas and targets

As well as identifying the five key areas, the White Paper[1] also focuses on the importance of healthy alliances and healthy settings within and across the key areas in taking forward work to achieve the specific targets.

For CHD and stroke, action is identified in the areas of smoking, diet, raised blood pressure, alcohol misuse and physical activity.

Four specific cancers are identified - breast, cervix, skin and lung. In the case of cervical and breast cancer the action builds on the already well-established screening programmes; for lung cancer new areas for action, such as reduction of smoking in pregnancy, are identified. The increasing problem of skin cancer is recognised.

Mental illness is being addressed by improving the information available on prevalence and outcomes of mental illness, the development of a comprehensive system of psychiatric services and the development of good practice in both primary and secondary care.

Action in HIV/AIDS and sexual health centres around encouraging the adoption of safe patterns of sexual behaviour among, and better family planning services for, young people. This will be important both for HIV/AIDS issues and other sexually transmitted diseases, and should reduce unplanned pregnancies. Needle-sharing among drug misusers is also identified as a topic for future action.

For accidents, three specific age-groups are targeted. Action in this key area will be particularly focused on the establishment of local alliances among many different organisations, which will work together to achieve reductions in accident mortality.

Second order priorities

Possible areas suggested during consultation but not included in the White Paper fell into three broad categories: those where there were already good existing initiatives, for which progress needed to be sustained and built on (eg childhood immunisation); areas where further research and development were needed (eg asthma and back pain); and areas where work was being taken forward through other mechanisms (eg diabetes mellitus, where targets had been set in the 1989 St Vincent's declaration[29]).

Implementation

Mechanisms have been set up to oversee the implementation and development of the strategy for health[1]. This includes the establishment of a Cabinet Committee chaired by the Lord President of the Council and three working groups with wide representation looking at different aspects of the strategy's implementation.

The way ahead

Much has been done to take forward the White Paper's[1] message. Management summaries, summaries for the general population and a cassette version for blind and partially-sighted people were produced and guidance was issued to the NHS (*First Steps for the NHS*[30]) which outlined action for the NHS to take in 1993/94. The 'Health at Work in the NHS' initiative was launched to look at how the NHS itself can ensure a safer, healthier working environment. Work is in hand to produce guidance on health promotion in the workplace, development of healthy alliances, and policy appraisal and health. However, it is crucial that the strategy is monitored and reviewed regularly. Much of this work will be taken forward by DH's Central Health Monitoring Unit and one of its first tasks was to produce the *Specification of National Indicators*[31], which gave full background information to health authorities on the White Paper targets[1] and the methods by which they would be monitored at national level. Publication of the White Paper[1] is only the beginning of a dynamic strategy which will be regularly monitored and reviewed, and built on when appropriate. It is important to have commitment from everyone to achieve the major health gains aimed for in this strategy.

HEALTH OF MEN

More boys than girls are born (the ratio is now 105:100), but males have a consistently higher mortality. The higher death rate among males is seen across all age-groups: infant mortality is 20% higher in boys than girls, and an 18-year-old man has an 80% chance of survival to 65 years, compared with an 88% chance for an 18-year-old woman. A better understanding of the reasons that underlie this higher mortality among males may be of benefit to men and women alike. About two-thirds of the male population in England in 1991 were men aged 15-64 years; demographic patterns over the past 10 years show an 11% increase in the numbers of young men aged 30-44 years, reflecting the ageing of so-called 'baby-boom' cohorts.

Mortality

Although the differences in mortality between men and women are the main topic of this chapter, it is important to remember that the main causes of death in men and women are similar. Nevertheless, accidents and suicide are particularly important causes of death among men under the age of 45 years.

Morbidity

Men have lower general practitioner (GP) consultation rates but higher hospital admission rates for diseases such as CHD and stroke.

Illnesses of men

Prostatism and cancer of the prostate: The incidence of prostatic hyperplasia and of prostate cancer increases with age. Different forms of treatment for both conditions are under evaluation.

Testicular tumours: Testicular tumours are the most common form of cancer in men aged 20-34 years. Mortality with current treatment is low but the incidence of testicular cancer has risen over the last decade.

X-linked disorders: Certain diseases are seen almost exclusively in men because of inheritance via the X chromosome: these diseases include haemophilia, Duchenne and Becker muscular dystrophy, and X-linked retinitis pigmentosa.

Male infertility: In about a quarter of couples investigated for infertility the man is found to be infertile because of deficient sperm production or abnormal sperm structure or motility. The cumulative success of donor insemination is 75%, but there is currently little effective treatment for most causes of male infertility; research continues into potential new treatments.

Impotence: Whilst most cases of impotence arise from psychological causes, physical causes should always be looked for and excluded.

HIV/AIDS and other sexually transmitted diseases: Up to the end of 1992, 93% of people with a diagnosis of AIDS and 88% of those infected with HIV were male. Over the past decade, HIV infection has emerged as a substantial contributor to male mortality (particularly among men aged 25-44 years) in the four Thames health Regions. For many other sexually transmitted diseases, the number of cases in men exceed those in women, although this difference may partly reflect the increased likelihood of symptoms appearing in men.

Mental health: Striking sex differences are seen in the incidence and prevalence of symptoms of mental disorders. Compared with women, men seem to be less likely to suffer neurotic symptoms but equally likely to suffer from psychotic disorders. For schizophrenia the peak onset in males occurs at a much earlier age (15-24 years) than in females (35-39 years). Although women are more likely to become depressed or to commit acts of deliberate self harm, men are twice as likely to die from suicide: this discrepancy is increasing, particularly among people aged 15-34 years.

Accidents: Over 75% of deaths caused by accidental injuries in the age range 15-64 years were in men. The causes of accidents differ: motor vehicle traffic accidents accounted for almost half of the accidental deaths in men, whereas accidental falls were the commonest cause in women.

Men, health and society

The majority of drug misusers notified to the Home Office are men, and more men than women are reported to be heavy drinkers. The social impact of financial problems, marital and family difficulties and homelessness, and associated drug and alcohol misuse, can be particularly high among men.

Health and work

Accidents at work are seen far more commonly among men (eg 98% of fatal injuries and 75% of major injuries) than in women. Studies of unemployed men indicate that unemployment may have an adverse effect on health even after adjustment for social class and pre-existing morbidity[32,33].

Improving the health of men

Although many men and women die from similar causes, there are clear gender differences in mortality and morbidity. Many causes of death and illness in men are potentially preventable, and health professionals and society as a whole need to change the behaviour of men to ensure that they achieve a similar life expectancy to women, as well as a high quality of life.

HEALTH CARE

Needs, effectiveness and outcomes

Assessing health care needs: During 1992, further epidemiologically based health needs reviews were published about stroke, renal disease, dementia, mental illness, prostatectomy for benign prostatic hyperplasia, varicose vein treatment, CHD, cancer of the lung, learning disabilities, hernia repair and cataract surgery. More are planned.

Basic sources of information: New and evolving information initiatives considerably enhanced the ability to collect, process, analyse and interpret key health data. Work on several health surveys has been started or completed during 1992 and the expanded Health Survey for England will start in January 1993.

National confidential enquiries: The purpose of a confidential enquiry is to improve understanding of the factors relating to a particular health outcome, and of how the risks of an unfavourable outcome might be reduced, if not avoided. Three new national confidential enquiries were established in 1992; like the two existing enquiries, they should make significant contributions towards improved outcomes.

Quality of service and effectiveness of care: The programme of clinical audit continues and is becoming established as a key part of NHS services. The Chief Medical and Nursing Officers jointly established the Clinical Outcomes Group to bring together work on clinical audit and outcomes of care: patients and the public are represented by two lay members.

Outcomes of care: Progress with central initiatives to develop health outcomes assessment during 1992 included creation of a database and the start of services by the United Kingdom (UK) Clearing House on Outcomes, the report of the Faculty of Public Health Medicine on the first phase of a feasibility study of population health outcome indicators, commissioning of the University of Surrey to analyse a first set of indicators, and substantial progress in the Central Health Outcomes Unit's preparation of a structured programme for the development of technical systems to assess health outcomes.

Primary health care

Effects of the new contract: 1992 was a year of consolidation. Progress included increased achievement of targets, action to support and to focus health promotion activity on national priorities, computerisation and developments in team working.

Strategy for health: Events during the year should lead to better targeted health promotion. Other projects begun in 1992 include a community-oriented primary care programme to encourage GPs to look at the overall health of their practice population.

Prescribing: The prescribing bill continued to rise alarmingly, with no convincing evidence of increased health gain: a Prescribing Task Force has been established to investigate the reasons for this increase. Other support continues for prescribers and a new information system (PACTLINE) is in use.

Clinical Audit: Clinical audit is becoming an established part of primary care. Multidisciplinary audit by all members of the primary health care team, and other carers, is being encouraged.

GP fundholding: GP fundholding is a driving force in the NHS reforms and is helping to provide a wider range of local services to patients.

Professional development: All members of the primary health care team must continue their professional development and training to achieve satisfactory standards of care in a changing world.

The way ahead: Medical advances mean that more complex treatments can now be provided in the community. Primary health care professionals need new skills for preventive care and to deal with changing patterns of disease.

Hospital services

Supra-Regional Services: During 1992, Supra-Regional status was designated for proton treatment of large uveal melanomas, a further heart transplantation unit at Queen Elizabeth Hospital, Birmingham, and a further liver transplantation unit at Freeman Hospital, Newcastle. Spinal injury services left the Supra-Regional arrangements. There was a striking increase in the number of enquiries from provider units about the mechanism to apply for Supra-Regional status.

Access and availability: During 1992 the Clinical Standards Advisory Group continued to act as an independent source of expert advice to Health Ministers and the NHS on standards of clinical care and access to and the availability of selected specialist services. A series of reports will be published from the Summer of 1993.

Cancer: In 1992, DH provided £20 million for diagnostic equipment and linear accelerators. Continuous hyperfractionated accelerated radiotherapy is being assessed and a new Minimum Data Set for cancer registration will be introduced in 1993.

Palliative care: The National Council for Hospices and Specialist Palliative Care Services co-ordinates the policies of charitable organisations and NHS units. At a European conference held in London, the Standing Medical and Standing Nursing and Midwifery Advisory Committees' report[34] on principles and provision of palliative care was presented.

Diabetes mellitus

In July 1992, a joint DH and British Diabetic Association Task Force was set up to advise on the implementation of the recommendations of the St Vincent Declaration on Diabetes Care and Research[29]. The Task Force will report on the priorities for further action in 1993.

Osteopathy

Mr Malcolm Moss MP introduced a Private Members' Bill, which seeks to establish a General Osteopathic Council, to the House of Commons in June 1992.

Mental health

Care Programmes, Specific Grant, and central London homeless mentally ill initiative: The funding of the Mental Illness Specific Grant was increased by 9% to £34.4 million, and by the end of 1992 the third phase of the Homeless Mentally Ill Initiative for homeless people sleeping rough in central London included four specialist hostels and five multidisciplinary community psychiatric teams.

Development of brief rating scales: In support of the first target in the mental illness key area of strategy for health, the Royal College of Psychiatrists was commissioned to lead the multidisciplinary development of brief rating scales to measure health, social functioning and quality of life.

OPCS psychiatric morbidity pilot: DH commissioned OPCS to carry out a national psychiatric morbidity survey to provide baseline data on the prevalence of mental illness in the population, its associated disabilities and risk factors, and use of services. A pilot study in 1992 demonstrated the feasibility and acceptability of the methodology, and a large scale study will start in 1993.

Mental health and primary care: Primary care provides considerable opportunities for prevention of mental illness. Prompt detection and treatment will improve outcome. DH has funded a number of initiatives to improve the detection and management of mental illness in primary care.

Occupational mental health: The importance of mental health in occupational settings was emphasised, with the mental health of the NHS workforce included as one of six national priorities in the NHS research and development programme of mental health research. In November, DH had a stand and held a breakfast hosted by Baroness Cumberlege to promote the strategy for health and mental health in the workplace at the national conference of the Confederation of British Industry.

Services for people with severe mental illness: The implementation of the Care Programme Approach, introduced in 1991 to provide a 'safety-net' for people with severe mental illness, was evaluated. A mental health Task Force under the leadership of Mr David King has been set up to develop local services, including psychosocial treatments that involve early intervention and skills training.

Services for mentally disordered offenders: The joint Home Office/DH review of services for mentally disordered offenders and others requiring similar services was completed in July 1992 and its final summary report[35] was published in November 1992. Responses to consultation papers overwhelmingly supported the direction of development proposed by its 276 recommendations.

Progress has been made with court diversion schemes, needs assessments, and funding for the provision of medium secure units. A new advisory committee on mentally disordered offenders will be established to follow up the review.

Maternity and child health services

Health Select Committee Reports on maternity services: The Health Committee's 1992 report[36] on maternity services proposed that a more user-friendly service should be developed. The Government's response[37] welcomed the proposal but noted the need to ensure safety for mother and baby.

Family planning services: Concern about the continuing high level of unintended pregnancies resulted in family planning services being selected as a key area of the strategy for health[1]. A target to reduce the rate of conceptions among girls under 16 years-of-age by at least 50% by the year 2000 was set. Regional Health Authorities (RHAs) reviewed their family planning services.

Cervical cancer screening: Cervical cancer is included in the cancer key area of the strategy for health[1]. Further improvement in screening coverage has been achieved, which should help to ensure that the target of reducing the incidence of invasive cervical cancer by 20% by the year 2000 is reached.

The Human Fertilisation and Embryology (Disclosure of Information) Act 1992: This Act[38] effected a small change in the confidentiality of information requirements of the Human Fertilisation and Embryology Act 1990[39].

Confidential Enquiry into Stillbirths and Deaths in Infancy: The National Advisory Body was established early in 1992 to steer the Confidential Enquiry into Stillbirths and Deaths in Infancy.

Sudden infant death syndrome: In 1991, an expert group gave initial advice on the relation of sleeping position of infants to cot death, and this was followed by the national campaign *Back to Sleep*. A key part of the advice was that the risk of cot death can be reduced if babies are not placed prone when laid down to sleep. Although the incidence of cot death had been falling prior to the campaign, the subsequent fall has been significantly greater.

Prophylaxis against vitamin K deficiency bleeding in infants: Newborn babies have been given prophylactic vitamin K, either intramuscularly or orally, to prevent vitamin K deficiency bleeding. During 1992, there was a report of a possible association between vitamin K given intramuscularly and the development of cancer in childhood[40,41,42]. The available facts did not permit a clear consensus on the safest form of prophylaxis for newborn babies[43], and the Chief Medical and Nursing Officers wrote to health professionals to set out the background to this debate and to provide guidance on the professional issues that had been raised[44].

Review of adoption law: The working group reviewing adoption law reported to

Ministers in July 1992[45]. Its recommendations were based on the principle that the child's welfare is paramount in decisions relating to adoption. After wide consultation the Government intends, when Parliamentary time permits, to introduce new legislation.

Learning disabilities

In October, Health Service Guidelines[46] and a Local Authority Circular[47] defined the health and social components of care. A shortfall in medium secure services for offenders with learning disabilities was identified by a DH/Home Office Review[48].

Disability and rehabilitation

1992 saw the selection of sites to participate in the Department's brain injury initiative; publication of a National Audit Office report on health services for physically disabled people aged 16 to 64 years; a conference on 'Disability, Teamwork and Independence'; the identification of rehabilitation as a candidate for future key area status in the strategy for health; and an increase in the number of doctors working in rehabilitation medicine.

Prison health care

The former Prison Medical Service was relaunched in May 1992 as the Health Care Service for Prisoners. The Directorate of Health Care and the Health Advisory Committee, chaired by Sir Donald Acheson, are committed to the concept of healthy prisons and to an increased emphasis on health promotion programmes for prisoners. The Health Care Service for Prisoners is seeking to become more closely aligned to the NHS and to become primarily a purchaser, rather than a provider, of health care services.

Health of elderly people

The number of very old people will increase in the next decade. Their needs will become an increasingly important factor in programmes designed to safeguard and improve the health of the population. Health promotion and prevention measures are as successful in older men and women as in younger people, and implementation of the strategy for health will improve the quality of life of older people as well as younger people. As a result of improved life expectancy, increasing numbers of frail older people now live in the community, either with a carer or on their own; effective collaboration between local authority social services departments and health authorities is essential.

Health of black and ethnic minority groups

The health of black and ethnic minority groups was the subject of the special chapter in last year's Report[49]. During 1992, the Secretary of State for Health chaired a working group on ethnic minority employment in the NHS, and Baroness Cumberlege was asked to take responsibility for improvements to the NHS services received by ethnic groups. Results from the ethnicity question included in the 1991 census showed that 6.2% of people in England are from black and ethnic minority backgrounds. DH supported the production of a wide range of materials that covered many issues affecting various minority groups; these provided information to the public, to patients and to health care professionals alike. DH also supported several conferences that highlighted ethnic minority health issues. Research programmes were set up to improve our knowledge of ethnicity and health, and the Standing Medical Advisory Committee Working Party on sickle cell disorder and thalassaemia continued its work. During the year there was particular concern about a rise in the suicide rate among young Asian women.

COMMUNICABLE DISEASES

HIV infection and AIDS

During 1992, the picture of the HIV/AIDS epidemic in England remained similar to the previous two years. Infection transmitted by sex between men still predominates among known AIDS patients and those reported positive for HIV, but an increasing proportion of known infections are found in people infected (mostly abroad) through heterosexual sex. The epidemic still seems to be concentrated in the London area.

HIV/AIDS and sexual health form one of the key areas in the Government's strategy for health White Paper[1]. Throughout 1992, DH continued support for public education through the Health Education Authority (HEA) and the National AIDS Helpline. The wider emphasis on sexual health has been reflected in educational and health promotion initiatives at both national and local level, and there have been further initiatives to target specific populations and to take account of different cultures and needs.

Other sexually transmitted diseases

The total number of new cases seen at genito-urinary medicine (GUM) clinics increased by 10%. This reflected an increase in viral sexually transmitted diseases (STDs), including HIV/AIDS, and in cases in which no STD was diagnosed. Reports of most non-viral STDs fell although some, such as gonorrhoea, show signs of reaching a plateau.

Immunisation

Immunisation coverage is now higher than ever before and many Districts are already reaching 1995 targets for all childhood vaccines. Notification of matching diseases remains at record low levels.

In September 1992, based on concerns about higher than previously appreciated risks of mumps virus meningitis, measles, mumps and rubella (MMR) vaccines containing the Urabe mumps strain were replaced with MMR II vaccine. This brand, containing Jeryl Lynn mumps strain, does not appear to be associated with mumps virus meningitis.

In October 1992, immunisation was introduced against *Haemophilus influenzae* type b (Hib) infection. Children now receive Hib vaccine at the same time as routine immunisations at 2, 3, and 4 months, and children who have commenced immunisation but who are under 4 years-of-age are also being immunised. The introduction of Hib vaccine has been supported by an information campaign for health professionals and a publicity campaign for the public.

Hepatitis C

Screening and supplementary tests for evidence of hepatitis C in blood donations continue to be refined.

Legionellosis

Reported cases of Legionnaires' disease increased from the record low of 1991, but there were still no major outbreaks.

Influenza

It was a quiet year for influenza. For the first time, the vaccines used within the EC were harmonised.

Tuberculosis

Notifications of tuberculosis increased by more than 5% compared with the previous year, a trend seen in many European countries.

Shigellosis

The increase in notifications of *Shigella sonnei* infection which occurred at the end of 1991 continued into 1992, but then gradually declined.

Travel-related disease

Three vaccines were added to those available for travellers, but most illness among people who travel abroad continues to be caused by diseases for which established vaccines are not available.

ENVIRONMENTAL HEALTH AND TOXICOLOGY

United Nations Conference on Environment and Development

The United Nations Conference on Environment and Development (UNCED) was held in June 1992 in Rio de Janeiro. Agreement was reached on an action programme for sustained development into the next century (Agenda 21), which includes proposals for the protection and promotion of health and for increased international work on chemical risk assessment and management. The International Programme on Chemical Safety (IPCS), to which the DH already makes a substantial contribution, will play a central role in this activity.

Chemical and physical agents in the environment

Small Area Health Statistics Unit: The Small Area Health Statistics Unit was set up to investigate ill-health, specifically mortality by cause and cancer incidence around point sources of environmental pollution. During 1992 the Unit investigated specific industrial installations, undertook point source enquiries and pursued methodological developments.

Air pollution episodes: The conclusions and recommendations[50] of the Advisory Group on the Medical Aspects of Air Pollution Episodes about sulphur dioxide, acid aerosols and particulates were accepted, and information is available on a telephone Helpline. The Group has nearly completed a study of the oxides of nitrogen. The Committee on the Medical Effects of Air Pollutants was established and is advising on possible relations between asthma and air pollution.

Effects of ultraviolet irradiation: The incidence of skin cancer is rising, probably from a combination of occupational and recreational exposure to ultraviolet radiation. To halt the year-on-year increase in incidence of skin cancer by the year 2005 is a target of the strategy for health[1].

Foodborne and waterborne diseases

The Advisory Committee on the Microbiological Safety of Food advised the Government on a definition of food poisoning for use throughout the UK, which was accepted and promulgated to all doctors in England and Wales in September 1992[51]. The Committee also completed its work on vacuum packaging and associated processes and on salmonella in eggs, and set up Working Groups on verocytotoxin-producing *Escherichia coli* (VTEC) and poultry meat. A study of infectious intestinal disease in England was commissioned at the end of the year, under the auspices of the Steering Group on the Microbiological Safety of Food.

The Steering Group on the Microbiological Safety of Food started to plan a large-scale study of infectious intestinal disease in England at the end of the year. Statutory notifications of food poisoning increased in 1992 compared with the previous three years. Reports of salmonellosis, campylobacter enteritis and infections caused by VTEC also increased. However, reports of listeriosis remain at a low level.

Only a small number of outbreaks of waterborne diseases were reported. A number of seminars and workshops were held on the importance of close liaison between District Health Authorities (DHAs), local authorities and water companies when handling waterborne outbreaks.

During the UK Presidency of the European Community (EC) a common position was agreed on the draft Directive on the Hygiene of Foodstuffs.

Toxicological safety

Working Party on Dietary Supplements and Health Foods: The Committee on Toxicity of Chemicals in Food, Consumer Products and the Environment (COT) was asked to review the safety in use of certain herbal substances. Comfrey was the first of these substances to be assessed. COT advised that only comfrey teas and tinctures should continue to be available to the public.

Dioxins in milk: DH continued to provide advice on dioxin contamination of three farms in Bolsover, particularly on the health risks from the levels of dioxins in meat and milk from these farms and on the results of blood tests for dioxins in individuals living on them.

Food carcinogen prioritisation: During 1992, work started on a scheme to prioritise chemical contaminants in food according to the carcinogenic risks which they pose to the population.   The scheme will rely heavily on the expertise of the Committees on the Carcinogenicity and the Mutagenicity of Chemicals in Food, Consumer Products and the Environment (COC and COM).

Advisory Committee on Novel Foods and Processes: The withdrawal from the market of germanium 'health' supplements continued, following the Committee's advice, and research into the aetiology of germanium nephrotoxicity was started. The Committee advised on the safety of two other health foods and a novel surveillance system to scan food cargoes.

Pesticide residues in food: In 1992, Government Departments started to frame revised regulations to introduce Maximum Residue Levels (MRLs) for a number of pesticide/crop combinations not covered under previous regulations, and to revise MRLs where they had been set on inadequate data. Surveillance of pesticide residues in food showed that intakes of pesticides were well within acceptable daily intakes.

Veterinary drug residues in food: Regulations came into effect in 1992[52] to make MRLs for veterinary drugs legally enforceable. EC regulations also came into force in 1992 to set out a framework for the regulation of veterinary drugs used in food-producing animals.

Implants: DH set up an independent advisory group to review evidence for a possible association between silicone breast implants and autoimmune disease. No evidence was found to indicate a need to change current practice or policy, but data are limited; a national registry of patients with breast implants will be set up in 1993.

OTHER EVENTS OF INTEREST IN 1992

Medicines Control Agency

Role and performance: The Medicines Control Agency's (MCA's) role is to protect the public health by ensuring that all medicines for human use are safe, effective and of high quality. The Agency has met all its public health targets, reduced licensing times, eliminated backlogs and achieved Trading Fund status.

Control of UK clinical trials: Clinical trials are controlled by legislation to protect patients in whom new medicines are tested. The MCA is receiving more applications for clinical trials and improving its ability to monitor them.

Reclassification of Medicines from Prescription Only to Pharmacy status: The MCA revised guidance on reclassifying Prescription Only Medicines (POMs) to allow over-the-counter supply from pharmacies. Safety remains the criterion for deciding whether prescription control is needed.

Developments in the European Community: The UK had a leading role in the assessment of medicines through the current EC procedures and in the successful negotiation of proposals for the future licensing and control of medicines in the EC. The UK negotiated and implemented several other EC pharmaceuticals measures.

Medical devices

The Medical Devices Directorate (MDD) continued to monitor the safety and efficacy of medical devices. It operates a Manufacturer Registration Scheme, issues advice to the NHS on safety, efficacy and use of devices, runs a reporting system for device-related adverse incidents, and issued some 150 evaluations reports on a wide range of medical equipment during 1992. Implementation of EC Directives for statutory regulation of medical devices continues.

During 1992, MDD received over 2,700 reports of problems, investigated over 1,000 of these in depth, and issued 24 Hazard Circulars and 67 Safety Action Bulletins.

Bioethics

Local Research Ethics Committees: From 1 February 1992, Local Research Ethics Committees were set up in every District to advise NHS bodies on the ethical acceptability of research proposals involving human subjects.

Bioethics in Europe: The Council of Europe has been active in bioethics for over 15 years. In 1992, the Ad Hoc Committee on Bioethics (CAHBI) became the Steering Committee on Bioethics (CDBI).

Medical manpower and education

Junior doctors' hours: Good progress was made toward the targets set out in the 'New Deal' on junior doctors' hours[53]. At 31 August 1992 only 3,234 juniors remained contracted for more than 83 hours, a reduction of over 10,000 since September 1990.

'Achieving a Balance': The number of consultants grew by 2.8% annually over the period 1986 to 1991, including the effect of centrally funded initiatives.

Women doctors and their careers: Improvement of career opportunities for women doctors remains a priority, with the promotion of the Women in Surgical Training scheme, equal opportunities policies and flexible training schemes.

Flexible training: Progress has been made in improving flexible training opportunities for doctors.

New career structure for doctors in community child health: The Joint Working Party on Medical Services for Children reported in November with a recommendation for a unified medical career structure in child health[54].

Postgraduate and continuing medical education: During 1992, the postgraduate and continuing medical education arrangements were improved by a strengthened Regional infrastructure, agreement of a new funding system to protect training opportunities for hospital doctors, and the introduction of contract sessions for GP course organisers.

Working Group on Specialist Medical Training: The Working Group on Specialist Medical Training, chaired by the Chief Medical Officer, considered all aspects of this subject in the light of EC Directives, and will publish a report for consultation in the Spring of 1993.

Undergraduate medical and dental education: The Steering Group on Undergraduate Medical and Dental Education and Research will publish its third report early in 1993.

Medical Manpower Standing Advisory Committee: Planning the Medical Workforce[55], the first report of the Medical Manpower Standing Advisory Committee, was published in December.

The Tomlinson Report

Sir Bernard Tomlinson's *Report of the Inquiry into London's Health Service, Medical Education and Research* was published in October[56]. The Government's response, a policy document *Making London Better*, will be published early in 1993, and will set out the framework for an improved health service for Londoners.

Dental health

Dental health of the nation: The dental health of the nation continues to improve among children and adults, but careful monitoring of some trends among children is essential.

General dental services: The Secretary of State for Health set up a fundamental review of the system of dental remuneration[57], after evidence suggested that payments to dentists during 1991/92 were significantly higher than expected.

Community dental services: The role of the community dental services is being reviewed.

Hospital dental services: The number of new outpatient referrals to consultant clinics in the specialties of orthodontics, paedodontics and restorative dentistry rose during 1991/92, although there was a fall for oral surgery.

Continuing education and training for dentists: Further priority areas for postgraduate training were identified, and a pilot project was set up to develop and to evaluate computer-assisted learning projects.

Dental research: Dental research commissioned by DH included a survey into the diet and dental health of very young children and into glove wearing by dentists.

INTERNATIONAL HEALTH

Britain, Europe and health

The health challenges faced in the UK are also faced by many other European countries. Pooling knowledge and sharing experience should improve public health across the EC and the wider Europe.

European Community

EC Presidency health initiatives: The UK held the EC Presidency from 1 July 1992 until 1 January 1993. A number of initiatives were taken forward by the Health Council, including a framework for EC action on public health, a Resolution on communicable disease, a Memorandum on reducing smoking, and the promotion of health education.

Treaty on European Union (Maastricht): The Maastricht Treaty will give renewed impetus to strengthened co-operation between Member States and put public health initiatives on a sounder legal footing.

European Economic Area: The EC will strengthen its co-operation with the European Free Trade Association (EFTA) by formation of the European Economic Area, creating the world's largest single market.

The Council of Health Ministers: The Council of Health Ministers met twice during the year, under the Portuguese and then the UK Presidency.

EC/WHO/Council of Europe: An ad-hoc committee has been set up to look for ways to improve working relations between the Community, the World Health Organization (WHO) and the Council of Europe.

Echo: In May, DH published the first issue of its international newsletter, *Echo*.

Free movement of people: A Working Group chaired by the Chief Medical Officer examined EC law on specialist medical training. The EC Regulations which co-ordinate the health care schemes of the Member States continue to operate effectively.

'Europe Against Cancer': A special programme, 'Cancer Prevention and Health Promotion in the Workforce', was launched in 1992.

Smoking: The Health Council adopted a second Directive on tobacco labelling.

Elderly and disabled people: In December 1992, the Secretary of State for Health launched the 1993 'European Year of Older People and Solidarity between Generations' in the UK.

AIDS and HIV infection: AIDS is an increasing problem world-wide. The UK continues to support WHO's Global Programme on AIDS.

Pharmaceuticals: After agreement to the EC Directive on Future Systems and Patents, the Commission has decided not to move towards harmonisation of pharmaceutical pricing.

Medical devices: There are new Directives to regulate the safety and marketing of medical devices in the EC.

Research and information technology: DH continues to be involved in EC research.

Nutrition: Efforts have been made to implement the nutrition labelling Directive.

Food safety: One of the major successes of the UK Presidency was the agreement of a common position on the draft Directive on the Hygiene of Foodstuffs.

Relations with Central and Eastern Europe

The UK continued to foster links with Central and Eastern Europe and to offer assistance to health programmes during difficult times for these countries.

Council of Europe

DH continued to be actively involved in the Council of Europe's many activities in health and bioethics.

The Commonwealth

The tenth Commonwealth Health Ministers' Conference in Cyprus in October on Environment and Health was the first international gathering of Ministers on environmental issues since the Earth Summit in Rio.

WHO

European Regional Committee: September's WHO European Regional Committee acknowledged the enormous challenge facing the Region resulting from political changes in the continent and WHO's need to respond to the health demands of Central and Eastern Europe.

Executive Board: The Chief Medical Officer was asked to chair an Executive Board Working Group to look at the future policy and working methods of WHO.

World Health Assembly: The World Health Assembly considered the Second Evaluation of the Global Strategy for 'Health for All by the Year 2000' and the Eighth Report on world health. The UK promoted a Resolution to heighten the profile of nursing.

References

1. Department of Health. *The Health of the Nation: a strategy for health in England.* London: HMSO, 1992 (Cm. 1986).
2. Department of Health. *The Patient's Charter.* London: Department of Health, 1991.
3. Department of Health. *The Health of the Nation Key Area Handbook: coronary heart disease and stroke.* London: Department of Health, 1993.
4. Department of Health. *The Health of the Nation Key Area Handbook: cancers.* London: Department of Health, 1993.
5. Department of Health. *The Health of the Nation Key Area Handbook: mental health.* London: Department of Health, 1993.
6. Department of Health. *The Health of the Nation Key Area Handbook: HIV/AIDS and sexual health.* London: Department of Health, 1993.
7. Department of Health. *The Health of the Nation Key Area Handbook: accidents.* London: Department of Health, 1993.
8. NHS Management Executive. *Priorities and planning guidance 1994-95.* Leeds: Department of Health, 1993 (Executive Letter: EL(93)54).
9. NHS Management Executive. *Local Target Setting: a discussion paper.* Heywood (Lancashire): Department of Health, 1993 (Executive Letter: EL(93)56).
10. Department of Health. *Working Together for Better Health.* London: Department of Health, 1993.
11. Department of Health. *Ethnicity and Health: a guide for the NHS.* Heywood (Lancashire): Department of Health, 1993.
12. Office of Population Censuses and Surveys. *Health Survey for England 1991.* London: HMSO, 1993.
13. Department of Health. *AIDS-HIV Infected Health Care Workers: guidance on the management of infected health care workers.* London: Department of Health, 1993.
14. UK Health Departments. *AIDS-HIV Infected Health Care Workers: practical guidance on notifying patients. Recommendations of the Expert Advisory Group on AIDS.* London: Department of Health, 1993.
15. Report of a Working Group. The incidence and prevalence of AIDS and other severe HIV disease in England and Wales for 1992-1997: projections using data to the end of June 1992. *Commun Dis Rep* 1993; **3 (Suppl 1)**: S1-17.
16. Department of Health. *Hospital Doctors: Training for the Future: the Report of the Working Group on Specialist Medical Training.* Heywood (Lancs): Department of Health, 1993. Chair: Dr Kenneth Calman.
17. Department of Health and Social Security. *On the State of the Public Health: the annual report of the Chief Medical Officer of the Department of Health and Social Security for the year 1987.* London: HMSO, 1988; 69-73.
18. Department of Health. *On the State of the Public Health: the annual report of the Chief Medical Officer of the Department of Health for the year 1988.* London: HMSO, 1989; 174-5.
19. Department of Health. *On the State of the Public Health: the annual report of the Chief Medical Officer of the Department of Health for the year 1989.* London: HMSO, 1990; 130-1.
20. Department of Health. *On the State of the Public Health: the annual report of the Chief Medical Officer of the Department of Health for the year 1990.* London: HMSO, 1991; 171-2.
21. Department of Health. *On the State of the Public Health: the annual report of the Chief Medical Officer of the Department of Health for the year 1991.* London: HMSO, 1992; 122-4.
22. North C, Ritchie J. *Factors Influencing the Implementation of the Care Programme Approach.* London: HMSO, 1993.
23. *National Health Service and Community Care Act 1990.* London: HMSO, 1990.
24. Allied Dunbar National Fitness Survey. *A report on activity patterns and fitness levels commissioned by the*

Sports Council and the Health Education Authority: main findings. London: Sports Council, 1992.

25. Department of Health. *The Nutrition of Elderly People.* London: HMSO, 1992 (Report on Health and Social Subjects no. 43).

26. Department of Health. *Folic acid and the prevention of neural tube defects.* Heywood (Lancashire): Department of Health, 1992.

27. White A, Freeth S, O'Brien M. *Infant Feeding 1990.* London: HMSO, 1992.

28. Department of Health. *The Health of the Nation: a consultative document for health in England.* London: HMSO, 1991 (Cm. 1523).

29. Diabetes Mellitus in Europe: a problem at all ages in all countries: a model for prevention and self care: a meeting organised by WHO and IDF Europe: proceedings. *Giornale Italiano di Diabetologia* 1990; **10** (Suppl).

30. NHS Management Executive. *First steps for the NHS: recommendations of the Health of the Nation focus groups.* London: Department of Health, 1992.

31. Department of Health. *Specification of National Indicators.* London: Department of Health, 1992.

32. Moser K, Goldblatt PO, Fox J, Jones DR. *Unemployment and mortality.* In: Goldblatt P, ed. *Longitudinal study 1971-1981: mortality and social organisations.* London: HMSO, 1990: 82-96.

33. Moser K, Goldblatt PO, Fox AJ, Jones DR. Unemployment and mortality: comparison of the 1971 and 1981 longitudinal study census samples. *BMJ* 1987; **294**: 86-90.

34. Standing Medical Advisory Committee/Standing Nursing and Midwifery Advisory Committee. *The principles and provision of palliative care.* London: HMSO, 1992.

35. Department of Health, Home Office. *Final Summary Report. Review of health and social services for mentally disordered offenders and others requiring similar services.* London: HMSO, 1992 (Cm. 2088).

36. House of Commons. Health Committee. *Maternity Services: second report from the Health Committee. Session 1991-92.* London: HMSO, 1992. Chair: Nicholas Winterton (HC 29; vol I).

37. Department of Health. *Government response to the second report of the Health Committee. 1991-92 session: maternity services.* London: HMSO, 1992 (Cm. 2018).

38. *Human Fertilisation and Embryology Act 1990.* London: HMS0, 1990.

39. *Human Fertilisation and Embryology (Disclosure of Information) Act 1992.* London: HMSO, 1992.

40. Golding J, Birmingham K, Greenwood R, Mott M. Childhood cancer, intramuscular vitamin K, and pethidine given during labour. *BMJ* 1992; **305**: 341-6.

41. Draper GJ, Stiller CA. Intramuscular vitamin K and childhood cancer. *BMJ* 1992; **305**: 709.

42. Hull D. Vitamin K and childhood cancer. The risk of haemorrhagic disease is certain; that of cancer is not. *BMJ* 1992; **305**: 326-7.

43. British Paediatric Association. *Vitamin K Prophylaxis in Infancy. Report of an Expert Committee.* London: British Paediatric Association, 1992. Chair: Professor Sir David Hull.

44. Department of Health. *Prophylaxis against vitamin K deficiency bleeding in infants.* Heywood (Lancashire): Department of Health, 1992 (Professional letter: PL/CMO(92)20, PL/CNO(92)14).

45. Department of Health, Welsh Office. *Review of Adoption Law: Report to Ministers of an Interdepartmental Working Group.* London: Department of Health and Welsh Office, 1992. Chair: Rupert Hughes.

46. Department of Health. *Health services for people with learning disabilities (mental handicap).* Heywood (Lancashire): Department of Health, 1992 (Health Service Guidelines: HSG(92)42).

47. Department of Health. *Social care for adults with learning disabilities (mental handicap).* Heywood (Lancashire): Department of Health, 1992 (Local Authority Circular: LAC(92)15).

48. Official Working Group on Services for People with Special Needs. *Review of services for mentally disordered offenders and others requiring similar services: people with learning disabilities (mental handicap) or with autism.* London: Department of Health/Home Office, 1992.

49. Department of Health. *On the State of the Public Health: the Annual Report of the Chief Medical Officer of the Department of Health for the year 1991.* London: HMSO, 1992 ; 8-9, 54-77.

50. Department of Health. *Sulphur Dioxide, Acid Aerosols and Particulates: report of the advisory group on the medical aspects of air pollution episodes.* London: HMSO, 1992. Chair: Professor Stephen Holgate.

51. Department of Health. *Definition of food poisoning.* London: Department of Health, 1992 (Professional Letter: PL/CMO(92)14).

52. Ministry of Agriculture, Fisheries and Food, Department of Health, Scottish Home and Health Department, Welsh Office. *Animals, Meat and Meat Products (Examination for Residues and Maximum Residue Limits) Regulations 1991.* London: HMSO, 1991 (Statutory Instrument 1991: no. 2843).

53. Department of Health. *Hours of Work of Doctors in Training: the new deal.* London: Department of Health, 1991 (Executive Letter: EL(91)82).

54. NHS Management Executive/British Medical Association. *Report of the Joint Working Party on Medical Services for Children.* London: Department of Health, 1992.

55. Medical Manpower Standing Advisory Committee. *Planning the medical workforce.* Heywood (Lancashire): Department of Health, 1992. Chair: Professor Colin Campbell.

56. Department of Health, Department for Education. *Report of the Inquiry into London's Health Service, Medical Education and Research: presented to the Secretaries of State for Health and Education by Sir Bernard Tomlinson.* London: HMSO, 1992.

57. Department of Health. *Fundamental Review of Dental Remuneration: report of Sir Kenneth Bloomfield KCB.* London: Department of Health, 1992.

CHAPTER 1

VITAL STATISTICS

(a) Population size

The 1992 populations described or used to calculate rates/ratios in this chapter are projections forward to 1992 from estimates provisionally rebased on the 1991 Census results. Final figures for 1991 will become available in the Summer of 1993 and estimates for 1992 will be available in the Autumn of 1993.

The estimated resident population of England at 30 June 1992 was 48.2 million, an increase of about 160,000 (0.3%) compared with 1991. Most of the increase (135,000) was due to natural change (excess of births over deaths) rather than net inward migration.

(b) Age and sex structure of the resident population

Appendix Table A.1 shows how the sizes of populations in various age-groups have changed in the periods 1981-91 and 1991-92. The number of children under the age of 5 years is now fairly stable, after rising during the early 1980s as a result of an increase in births from the very low levels seen in the late 1970s. The population of children of school age (5-15 years) has also stabilised because the small late-1970s birth cohorts have reached younger working ages (16-44 years). The large 1960s birth cohorts, which had caused numbers in the younger working ages to rise between 1981 and 1991, are now beginning to increase numbers in the older working ages (45-64 years for men, 45-59 years for women). Recent large increases in the number of pensioners aged 75-84 years have now tailed off as survivors from the smaller cohorts born during World War I have begun to reach this age-group. However, the rapid increase in the number of people aged 85 years and over continues.

(c) Fertility statistics - aspects of relevance for health care

Total conceptions

Data on conceptions relate to pregnancies which led to a maternity or to a legal termination under the Abortion Act 1967[1]; they exclude spontaneous and illegal abortions. The date of conception is estimated to occur 38 weeks before the date of confinement. As many of the births and some of the abortions in 1992 were conceived during the previous year, the latest available data are for 1991 and are provisional. In 1991, an estimated 809,111 conceptions occurred to women resident in England, a 2% fall on the 1990 figure (see Table 1.1). Of these, 44% occurred outside marriage, compared with 29% in 1981. There has been a steady rise in the overall conception rate during the last decade. However, in 1991 it decreased to 78.1 per 1,000 women aged 15-44 years.

29

Table 1.1: Conceptions inside and outside marriage, England, 1981, 1990 and 1991

Age of woman	All conceptions			Inside marriage¹			Outside marriage²		
	1981	1990	1991†	1981	1990	1991†	1981	1990	1991†
*Under 16**									
Number	8106	8111	7368	52	31	26	8054	8080	7342
Rate	7.3	10.1	9.3	0.0	0.0	0.0	7.3	10.0	9.3
*Under 20***									
Number	108202	108037	96866	26011	10695	9432	82191	97342	87434
Rate	56.9	68.8	65.0	297.1	286.7	296.0	45.3	63.5	59.9
*All ages****									
Number	710534	825695	809111	507558	468567	455582	202976	357128	353529
Rate	72.6	79.6	78.1	86.1	85.0	83.6	52.2	73.5	72.0

* Rates per 1,000 female population aged 13-15 years.
** Rates per 1,000 female population aged 15-19 years.
*** Rates per 1,000 female population aged 15-44 years.
† Provisional.
1 Rates per 1,000 female married population within each age-group.
2 Rates per 1,000 female unmarried population within each age-group.

Source: OPCS

Total births

Table 1.2 shows there were 651,784 live births in England in 1992, 1% less than in 1991. Despite an upward trend over the past decade, this was the second successive year to show a fall. The total period fertility rate (TPFR) measures the average number of children that would be born per woman if the current age-specific rates continued throughout her childbearing years. It was 1.80 in 1992, compared with 1.82 in 1991. Since 1972 the TPFR for England has remained below 2.1, the level which would lead to the long-term 'natural' replacement of the population.

Whilst the overall number of live births decreased, births outside marriage increased between 1991 and 1992: they accounted for 31% of all live births in 1992, compared with 30% in 1991 and 14% in 1982. In 1992, over half of the births outside marriage were jointly registered by parents who were living at the same address, and presumably cohabiting.

Abortions

Based on provisional data, a total of 153,613 abortions were performed in 1992 under the Abortion Act 1967[1] on women who were resident in England. This represents a decrease of 6,576 (4%) compared with 1991, but an increase of 31,162 (25%) compared with 1982. Of the total, 89% were carried out at under 13 weeks gestation, and only 3% were performed beyond 16 weeks gestation.

In 1992, 31% of all abortions carried out on resident women were on those in their early 20s, whilst only 12% were on those aged 35 years and over. The abortion rate was highest among women aged 20-24 years (26.2 abortions per 1,000 women aged 20-24 years).

Conceptions and abortions to teenagers

The teenage conception rate per 1,000 women aged 15-19 years rose from 56.9 in 1981 to 65.0 in 1991, based on provisional data. The conception rate for females aged under 16 years was 9.3 per 1,000 girls aged 13-15 years, a decrease of 8% compared with 1990.

Based on provisional data, 19% of legal abortions in 1992 were on women aged under 20 years; of these, 10% were on girls aged under 16 years. Over the past decade abortions on women aged under 20 years have risen from 14.8 per 1,000 women aged 14-19 years in 1982 to 17.2 per 1,000 in 1992.

Contraception

Results from the 1991 General Household Survey (GHS) indicate that 45% of women aged 18-29 years used the contraceptive pill, while 45% of women aged 35 years and over (or their partners) were sterilised (see Table 1.3). The condom is the second most frequently used contraceptive method in both of these groups.

Table 1.2: Numbers of live births and live births outside marriage, crude birth rate, general and total period fertility rates, England, 1982, 1991 and 1992

Year of birth	Live births	Crude birth rate (births per 1,000 population of all ages)	General fertility rate (births per 1,000 women aged 15-44 years)	Total period fertility rate (TPFR)	Live births outside marriage		
					Solely registered	Jointly registered	
						Same address	Different address
1982	589711	12.6	59.7	1.75	34331	50857	
1991	660806	13.7	63.7	1.82	50844	109471	38623
1992	651784	13.6*	62.8*	1.80*	48312	113058	41055

* Provisional.

Note: The jointly registered same/different address data are unavailable before 1983.

Source: OPCS

Table 1.3: *Women aged 16-49 years: percentage using the contraceptive pill, sterilisation and condom as methods of contraception by age, Great Britain, 1991*

Current use of contraception	Age (years)								
	16-17	18-19	20-24	25-29	30-34	35-39	40-44	45-49	Total
Sterilisation	0	0	1	8	21	38	50	47	25
Pill	16	46	48	42	25	11	4	2	23
Condom	10	15	14	19	17	20	13	12	16
Total - at least one method	*22*	*55*	*65*	*73*	*75*	*79*	*78*	*70*	*70*
Total not using a method	78	45	35	27	25	21	22	30	30
Base = 100%*	267	260	758	931	956	753	857	789	5571

* Percentages do not add to totals because of rounding and because some women used more than one non-surgical method. Only the major non-surgical methods used are included in this table.

Source: OPCS

22% of women aged 16-17 years used contraception: 16% reported using the contraceptive pill, and 10% condoms, which suggests that some young couples may be using the pill and condom in combination.

First births within marriage and social class (as defined by husband's occupation)

The increase in mean maternal age at first birth within marriage has continued. In 1992 it was 27.8 years, over 2 years higher than in 1982 (see Table 1.4). This trend was reflected in all social classes (as defined by husband's occupation). A striking rise in births to women aged 30 years and over was seen in the last decade and this trend has continued in the early 1990s. Table 1.5 shows that the number of first births to these women was 5% higher in 1992 than in 1991, and over 60% higher than in 1982.

Table 1.4: *Mean age of women at first live birth within marriage, according to social class of husband, England, 1982, 1991 and 1992*

Social class of husband	Mean age of women at first birth within marriage (years)		
	1982	1991	1992
All social classes	25.5	27.5	27.8
I and II	27.8	29.0	29.2
III Non-manual	26.2	27.7	28.0
III Manual	24.7	26.7	27.1
IV and V	23.4	25.8	26.0
Other*	23.8	25.6	26.1

* Residual groups include members of the armed forces, students and those whose occupation was inadequately described.
Note: Figures for social class are based on a 10% sample.

Source: OPCS

33

Table 1.5: *First births within marriage to women aged 30 years and over, England, 1982, 1991 and 1992*

Age of mother (years)	Number of births (thousands)		
	1982	1991	1992
All ages 30 and over	31.4	49.1	51.7
30-34	25.2	38.6	40.2
35-39	5.6	9.3	10.0
40-44	0.6	1.2	1.4
45 and over	0.0	0.0	0.0

Note: 1982 figures for age-groups are based on a 10% sample.

Source: OPCS

Multiple births

The number of multiple births has risen steadily over the past decade, reaching 1.3% of all maternities in 1992. Of the 8,081 multiple maternities in 1992, 193 resulted in triplets or higher order births - a decrease of 4% compared with 1991, but about three times the number in 1982 (see Table 1.6). This rise over the past decade is thought to be largely due to an increase in the use of fertility drugs and other procedures to assist conception. Figures provided by the Human Fertilisation and Embryology Authority show that, in the United Kingdom, there were 75 triplet pregnancies conceived as a result of in-vitro fertilisation procedures in 1991. However, not all of these pregnancies would have resulted in registrable live births or stillbirths.

Reference

1. *Abortion Act 1967 (as amended by Statutory Instrument: SI 480c.10).* London: HMSO, 1991.

Table 1.6: *Maternities with multiple births, England, 1982, 1991 and 1992*

Year	Maternities with multiple births			Maternities with multiple births per 1,000 maternities
	All	Twins	Triplets or higher	
1982	5920	5854	66	10.1
1991	7940	7739	201*	12.1
1992	8081	7888	193	12.5

* Incorrectly quoted as 212 in last year's Report.

Source: OPCS

34

(d) Mortality

The number of deaths registered in England decreased from 533,972 in 1991 to 522,656 in 1992, a fall of 2.1%. The crude mortality rate fell from 11.1 per 1,000 population in 1991, to 10.8 per 1,000 in 1992.

Mortality rates 1982-92

Monitoring mortality during the 1980s has shown that, for most age and sex groups, death rates fell throughout the decade. However, mortality rates for men aged 15-44 years rose by 8% between 1985 and 1990, although since 1990 this rate has decreased by 4% (see Figures 1.1 and 1.2). The fall in mortality rates among those aged 75 years and over has slowed down, especially among women. Mortality rates among children have fallen dramatically since 1988 - by 24% and 21% among boys and girls, respectively. It should be noted that there is a slight discontinuity between 1991 and earlier years due to rebasing of population estimates on 1991 Census results.

Figure 1.1: *Percentage change in age-specific mortality for males, England, 1982-92 (1982 = 100)*

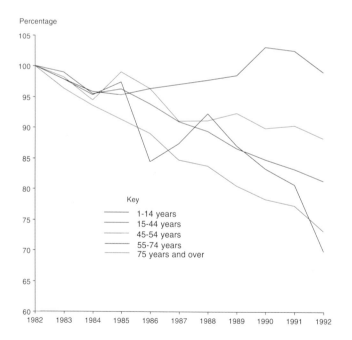

Source: OPCS

Figure 1.2: *Percentage change in age-specific mortality for females, England, 1982-92 (1982 = 100)*

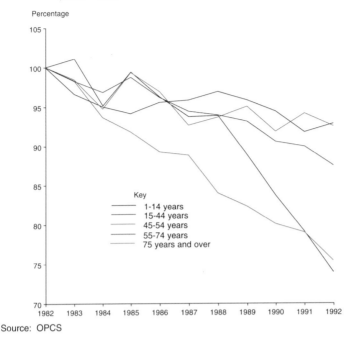

Percentage

Key
- 1-14 years
- 15-44 years
- 45-54 years
- 55-74 years
- 75 years and over

Source: OPCS

Trends in mortality in the 15-44 years age-group

A detailed analysis of excess deaths among young adults was summarised in the Report for 1990[1]. Data were combined for the years 1984-86, when death rates began to rise; these were compared with figures for the years 1987-89. A further comparison is now possible because 1990-92 data are available. As before, for women, death rates among those aged 40-44 years continued to decline in the same way as for those aged 45-54 years. The 5-year age-specific death rates for women aged 15-29 years remained the same, and those for women in their 30s decreased, having levelled off during the period 1984-89. For men, the death rate for those aged 40-44 years was very similar in the two periods. Each 5-year age-group of men between 20 and 39 years-of-age showed a rise in death rate. For men aged 15-19 years the rate in the years 1990-92 was similar to that in the period 1987-89.

An analysis of deaths in these 5-year age-groups has been carried out by main causes. The number of deaths occurring in the period 1990-92 was compared with the number expected based on 1987-89 cause-specific rates. The summary for men and women aged 15-39 years is shown in Table 1.7, alongside the previous summary which compared 1987-89 deaths with those in the period 1984-86. The picture for men is very similar to the analysis for 1987-89 deaths. Decreases in deaths from cancer, circulatory diseases and accidents continued, but were again more than offset by increased deaths from suicides, open verdict deaths and AIDS. Other increases, which may be AIDS-related, were recorded

36

for deaths from infections and nervous system and respiratory diseases. There was also a continuing increase in deaths from diseases of the digestive system, mostly accounted for by chronic liver disease.

Table 1.7: *Increases/decreases in numbers of deaths by cause, 1987-89, compared with expected numbers based on 1984-86 death rates, and 1990-92, compared with 1987-89, among men and women aged 15-39 years, England and Wales*

Cause of death (ICD 9 Codes)	Increase/decrease in number of deaths			
	Men		Women	
	1987-89/ 1984-86	1990-92/ 1987-89	1987-89/ 1984-86	1990-92/ 1987-89
Infectious and parasitic (001-139)	24	84	12	12
Cancer (140-208)	-159	-153	-158	-319
Breast (174)			7	-133
Cervix (180)			25	-102
Other			-190	-85
Nervous system (320-389)	46	19	55	3
Heart disease (410-429)	-173	-68	-58	30
Cerebrovascular disease (430-438)	-131	-55	-10	-65
Respiratory disease (460-519)	44	126	24	-83
Diseases of digestive system (520-579)	4	104	90	64
Congenital malformations (740-759)	-23	-5	3	3
Accidents (E800-E949)	-243	-107	-120	53
Suicide (E950-E959)	344	424	-87	5
Open verdict (E980-E989)*	476	234	147	-22
AIDS (279)**	307	225	24	30
Other causes	131	248	6	-31
Net change in deaths	647 (1376-729)	1076 (1464-388)	-72 (393-465)	-321 (200-521)

* Injury undetermined whether accidentally or purposely inflicted.

** ICD category 279 is 'Disorders involving the immune mechanism', most of which are AIDS.

Source: OPCS

There was a net decrease in deaths among women aged 15-39 years between the periods 1987-89 and 1990-92; this change was greater than that between the years 1984-86 and 1987-89. The pattern for cancer has changed, with breast and cervical cancer causing many fewer deaths in the period 1990-92 than expected from the rates in the period 1987-89. The increase in digestive system deaths, mainly chronic liver disease, continued.

Suicides and undetermined deaths

In 1992 there were 5,541 suicides and undetermined deaths in England, compared with 5,567 in 1991. The combined figure for suicides and undetermined deaths has remained at about the same level since 1982, but this apparent stability masks an increase in male deaths and a fall in female deaths.

The proportion of suicides and undetermined deaths accounted for by males has increased from 62% in 1982 to 73% in 1992. In 1992 there were 4,052 male suicides and undetermined deaths in England, 17% more than in 1982, whereas female suicides and undetermined deaths decreased from 2,084 in 1982 to 1,489 in 1992, a fall of 29%.

The remainder of this section describes deaths in England and Wales combined. The male suicide rate has been increasing since the early 1970s[2], due to an increasing rate among those aged 15-44 years. The female suicide rate has been decreasing since the mid-1960s, but less rapidly among those aged 15-44 years than for women aged 45 years and over.

Figure 1.3 compares regional percentage changes in suicide rates for men and women aged 15-44 years. The comparison is for the periods 1979-83 and 1985-89, and is shown for recorded suicides and for suicides and undetermined deaths combined. Rates of suicide and undetermined death in young men increased in all Regions: by far the largest increase, of 58%, occurred in East Anglia, with the smallest increases in North East and North West Thames - 3% and 4%, respectively. For young women, rates for suicide and undetermined death fell in all but three Regions: South East Thames, East Anglia and Oxford. North West Thames saw the largest decrease of 29%.

When the 15-44 years age-group is analysed by marital status, divorced and widowed men have the highest rates of suicide and undetermined death. In each 10-year age-group, apart from men aged 15-24 years, single, widowed and divorced men generally have rates which are about three times greater than those of married men. However, rates of suicide and undetermined death among married men increased between the years 1972-74 and 1987-89, whereas rates for divorced men decreased, and rates for single men (except those aged 15-24 years) generally stayed the same (see Figure 1.4). Over the same period the distribution of marital status in this population changed quite dramatically; in particular, the proportion of single and divorced men increased (see Figure 1.5). In the period 1972-74 the rate of suicide and undetermined death for men aged 15-44 years was 115 per million, rising to 186 per million in the period 1987-89. If there had been no changes in the proportions of men in different marital status groups, the rate in the period 1987-89 would have been 149 per million. This finding indicates that half of the increase in rates of suicide and undetermined death among young men over this period may be related to the smaller proportions who are married.

References

1. Department of Health. *On the State of the Public Health: the annual report of the Chief Medical Officer of the Department of Health for the year 1990.* London: HMSO, 1991; 34.
2. Charlton J, Kelly S, Dunnell K, Evans B, Jenkins R, Wallis R. Trends in suicide deaths in England and Wales. *Population Trends 69.* London: HMSO, 1992.

Figure 1.3: *Suicide deaths: percentage change in Regional death rates for men and women aged 15-44 years, England and Wales, 1979-83 to 1985-89*

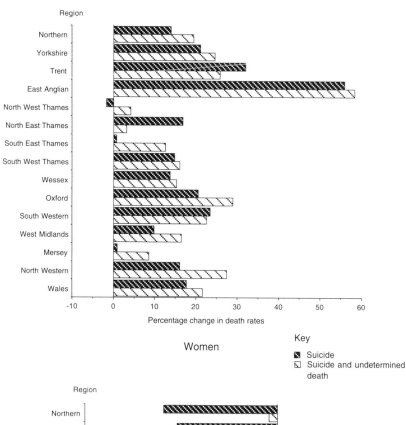

Men

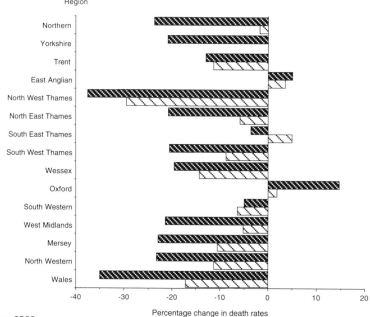

Women

Source: OPCS

Figure 1.4: *Suicide rates by sex and marital status for people aged 15-44 years, England and Wales, 1972-89*

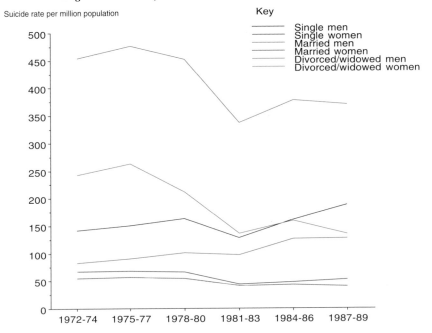

Source: OPCS

Figure 1.5: *Marital status of men and women aged 15-44 years, England and Wales, 1972 and 1989*

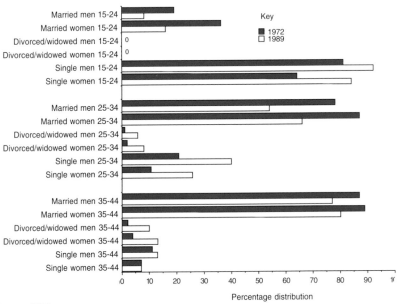

Source: OPCS

(e) Infant and perinatal mortality

Infant mortality

During 1992 in England, 4,259 babies died before the age of one year. Of these, 2,792 (66%) died in the neonatal period (under 28 days after live birth), and 1,467 (34%) in the post-neonatal period (from 28 days to under 1 year).

The infant mortality rate for England was 6.5 per 1,000 live births, the lowest ever recorded. This represents a fall of 11% from 7.3 per 1,000 live births in 1991 (see Figure 1.6). The neonatal mortality rate remained unchanged at 4.3 per 1,000 live births in 1992. Thus the fall in the overall infant mortality rate was due to a 25% decrease in the post-neonatal mortality rate, from 3.0 per 1,000 live births in 1991 to 2.3 in 1992. Most of the decrease in the latter can be accounted for by a 38% fall in the rate due to respiratory diseases (International Classification of Diseases [ICD] 9th Revision Chapter VIII), and of 50% in that due to sudden infant death syndrome (SIDS, ICD 798.0). The post-neonatal mortality rate due to SIDS has now fallen by 69% from its highest rate of 2.0 per 1,000 live births in 1988 to 0.6 in 1992. There were also 56 neonatal deaths attributed to SIDS during 1992.

Figure 1.6: *Deaths in the first year of life, England, 1982-92*

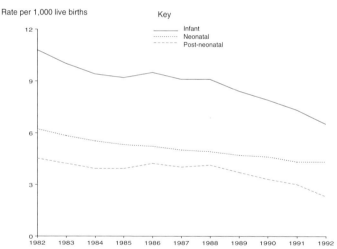

Source: OPCS

SIDS is only selected as the underlying cause of post-neonatal death when it is the sole cause mentioned on the death certificate. In 1992 there were another 37 post-neonatal deaths where SIDS, 'cot death', or some similar term was mentioned on the death certificate but was not selected as the underlying cause of death because another, more specific term had also been provided.

Perinatal mortality (stillbirths and deaths in the first week of life)

On 1 October 1992, the legal definition of a stillbirth was altered from a baby born dead after 28 completed weeks of gestation or more to one born dead after

41

24 completed weeks gestation or more. In 1992 in England there were 2,975 stillbirths, which included 198 stillbirths of between 24 and 27 completed weeks gestation that were registered between 1 October and 31 December 1992. The stillbirth and perinatal mortality rates were 4.5 and 7.9 per 1,000 total births, respectively - the lowest ever recorded. If the 198 stillbirths registered because of the change in legal definition are excluded, the stillbirth and perinatal mortality rates for 1992 would be even lower at 4.2 and 7.6 per 1,000 total births, respectively, and would represent falls of 8% and 6%, respectively, compared with the 1991 rates of 4.6 per 1,000 total births for stillbirths and 8.0 for perinatal mortality.

(f) Acute and chronic sickness

The GHS is a continuous survey collecting information about 20,000 adults and 5,000 children in Great Britain each year. It provides two measures of chronic sickness. Firstly, people are asked whether they have any long-standing illness, disability or infirmity. Those who answer "Yes" are then asked "What is the matter with you?", and then whether this limits their activities in any way. Acute sickness is measured by asking whether, in the two weeks before interview, people had to cut down on any of the things they usually do because of illness or injury. In 1991, 31% reported a long-standing illness, 18% a limiting long-standing illness and 12% restricted activity in the previous two weeks. Figure 1.7 shows trends from 1979 to 1991 for these three measures for males and

Figure 1.7: *Three-year moving averages of measures of morbidity from the General Household Survey, males and females, Great Britain, 1979-91*

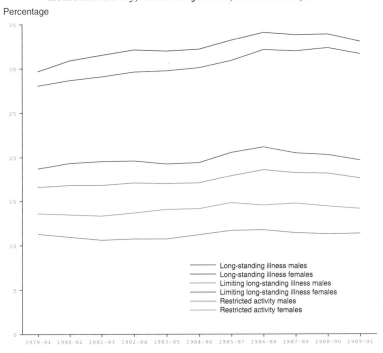

Source: OPCS

42

females, with the data presented as three-year moving averages to smooth out year-on-year fluctuations. The prevalence of acute sickness has changed little. The prevalence of reported long-standing illness increased during the 1980s. Towards the end of the decade the increase slowed, and then a slight fall occurred.

(g) Trends in cancer* incidence and mortality

Data from the 1988 and 1989 GHS show that 1% of adults reported cancer as a cause of long-standing illness. This estimate can be compared with that based on the Office of Population Censuses and Surveys (OPCS) Longitudinal Study, which is discussed in the report of the 1990 review of the cancer registration system[1]. The study brings together, for 1% of the population, information from the National Cancer Registration Scheme, successive Censuses and death registration. It suggests that just over half a million people alive in 1981 would have had a cancer registered in the preceding ten years - again a prevalence of around 1%.

The latest national (England and Wales) totals of cancer registrations relate to 1988. Appendix Tables A.7 and A.8 show the numbers registered by age, sex and site. Although trends over the period 1978-88 must be interpreted with caution, for all cancers together there was no change in incidence. However, when specific sites of malignancy are examined there are some trends of note.

When adjusted for age, the number of lung cancer registrations decreased for males but increased for females between 1978 and 1988. For both sexes there was an increase in the number of registrations of malignant melanoma of the skin in 1988 compared with 1987, and there was an overall increase during the period 1978-88. During the same period there was a decrease in the number of registrations of stomach cancer. There were marked downward trends for lymphosarcoma and reticulosarcoma and for Hodgkin's disease, but an upward trend for other malignant neoplasms of lymphoid and histiocytic tissue, to which less well specified lymphomas would be coded.

The upward trends for bladder cancer and malignant neoplasm of the kidney and other unspecified urinary organs between 1978 and 1984 appear to be levelling off for females. However, the situation is less clear for males. The number of registrations of carcinoma-in-situ of the cervix uteri was very much higher in 1984 than in previous years, which themselves showed an upward trend, and has continued to increase markedly. However, in respect of carcinoma-in-situ, possible improvements in the level of completeness of registration and in ascertainment need to be taken into account.

As with the incidence of all cancers, there has been no decline in mortality in recent years. Age-standardised death rates since the 1920s are shown in Figure 1.8. For males the post-war rise levelled off in the 1970s. For females there was a declining trend until the early 1960s, followed by a rise. Within these totals, however, there was a rise and then a fall in the rate for cancer of the

*cancer = malignant neoplasm

Figure 1.8: *Main types of cancer: age-standardised death rates per million population by sex, England and Wales, 1921-25 to 1991-92*

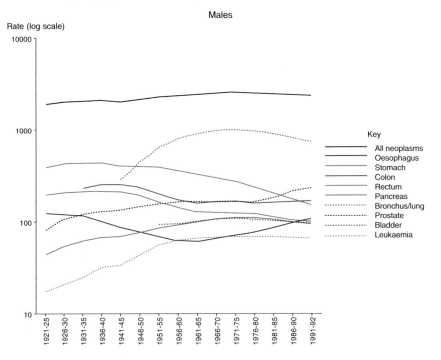

Males

Rate (log scale)

Key
All neoplasms
Oesophagus
Stomach
Colon
Rectum
Pancreas
Bronchus/lung
Prostate
Bladder
Leukaemia

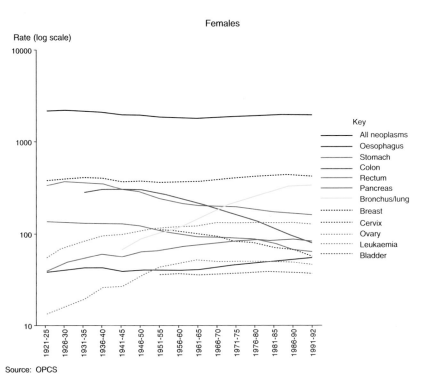

Females

Rate (log scale)

Key
All neoplasms
Oesophagus
Stomach
Colon
Rectum
Pancreas
Bronchus/lung
Breast
Cervix
Ovary
Leukaemia
Bladder

Source: OPCS

bronchus/lung in males, contrasting with a continuing rise in females. There was a steady fall in the rate for cancer of the stomach in both sexes.

Reference

1. Office of Population Censuses and Surveys. *Review of the national cancer registration system: report of the Working Group of the Registrar General's Medical Advisory Committee.* London: HMSO, 1990 (Series MB1 no. 17).

(h) Trends in reporting congenital malformations

Appendix Table A.6 shows that, according to provisional data for 1992, the rate for malformed live births in England decreased to 86.2 per 10,000 live births, 12% lower than in 1991 and 24% lower than in 1990. The rate for malformed stillbirths fell to 2.7 per 10,000 total births, 4% lower than in 1991 and 10% lower than in 1990.

An exclusion list was introduced in January 1990 to identify minor anomalies which should no longer be notified to OPCS. As a result, the total number of notifications received by OPCS fell by 4,058 (34%) between 1989 and 1990. This fall was accounted for entirely by a decrease in notifications of malformed live births. Three groups shown in the table were affected by the exclusion list: ear and eye malformations, cardiovascular malformations and talipes. For these three groups the comments in the following paragraphs are restricted to the changes that took place between 1990 and 1992; for the remainder the comments refer to the changes between 1980 and 1992.

Since 1980 there has been a marked reduction in the rate of central nervous system anomalies for live births (from 17.6 to 4.2 per 10,000 live births) and stillbirths (from 10 to 0.8 per 10,000 total births). Conditions such as hydrocephalus and anencephaly, which are within the group most likely to be detected prenatally by diagnostic ultrasound or alphafetoprotein screening, have shown the largest fall. A similar decrease has been reported in other countries[1].

The rates of hypospadias/epispadias and polydactyly/syndactyly per 10,000 live births have fallen by about one half and one quarter, respectively, since 1980; in 1992, the respective rates were 8.0 and 11.4. Since 1990, the rate of ear and eye malformations per 10,000 live births has fallen from 5.9 to 3.6, and that of talipes from 14.9 to 11.3. For cardiovascular malformations, the rate per 10,000 live births has decreased from 8.4 to 7.7, whilst the rate for stillbirths has fallen from 0.3 to 0.1 per 10,000 total births.

Reference

1. Sellers MJ. Unanswered questions on neural tube defects. *BMJ* 1987; **24**: 1-2.

(i) Appendix Tables and their content (pages 211-221)

Appendix Table 1: *Population age and sex structure, England, 1992, and changes by age, 1981-91 and 1991-92*

This table is described on the first page of this chapter.

Appendix Table 2: *Five main causes of death for males and females at different ages, England, 1992*

This table contrasts the major causes of mortality in different age-groups. It should be noted that the rankings are dependent on the particular groupings of disease chosen. At the age of 35 years and over, the major burden of mortality derives from circulatory diseases and malignant neoplasms. At ages 15-34 years, road vehicle accidents, other causes of injury and poisoning, and suicide are major contributors to death, particularly in males. These causes of death - other than suicides - are also important in childhood, although congenital anomalies and diseases of the nervous system and sense organs also rank highly.

Appendix Table 3: *Relative mortality from various conditions when presented as numbers of deaths and future years of 'working life' lost, England and Wales, 1992*

Data presented include the total number of deaths at all ages attributed to selected causes. The percentage distribution of the number of deaths demonstrates the major impact of circulatory disease and cancer in both sexes. In 1992, over 80% of deaths occurred at the age of 65 years and over.

Data are also presented for years of 'working life' lost between the ages of 15 and 64 years in order to indicate the impact of the various causes of death occurring at younger ages. For this tabulation, a death occurring under the age of 15 years accounts for the loss of the full 50-year period between the ages of 15 and 64 years, whereas death at age 60 years contributes a loss of only 5 years of 'working life'. Thus weight is given to the age at death as well as the number of deaths, and emphasis is given to the burden of deaths occurring at younger ages.

For males, although circulatory disease and cancer still contribute substantially to loss of 'working life', other causes become more prominent. These include accidents (mainly motor vehicle) and suicide, and also those deaths occurring early in life - particularly infant deaths, which account for about 15% of years of 'working life' lost. Current registration procedures preclude presentation of infant deaths occurring under the age of 28 days in this table, although figures for sudden infant death syndrome (SIDS) - for which about 6% of cases occur under the age of 28 days - have been included.

For females, the total years of future 'working life' lost from all causes combined is much less than for males, reflecting the considerably lower death rates in females. Cancer - particularly of the breast, cervix, uterus and ovary - is a major contributor to loss of life in females aged under 65 years. In 1992, cancer accounted for 22% of all female deaths, but 41% of years of 'working life' lost. By contrast, although causing 44% of the total number of deaths, circulatory disease accounted for only 15% of the years of future 'working life' lost. In other respects, the pattern is broadly similar to that for males, although accidents account for a smaller proportion of deaths among females.

Appendix Table 4: *Trends in 'avoidable' deaths, England and Wales, 1979-92*

The concept of 'avoidable' deaths was discussed in detail in the Report of 1987[1]. These indicators - developed in this country by Professor Walter Holland and his colleagues[2] - have been chosen to identify selected causes of mortality amenable to health service intervention, either preventive or curative. They might best be called 'potentially avoidable' deaths as, while it might not be possible to prevent every death deemed avoidable, it is expected that a substantial proportion could be prevented. The indicators are now published as part of the Public Health Common Data Set.

The table presents recent secular trends of nine categories of 'avoidable' deaths. The data are presented as age-standardised mortality ratios, which adjust for differences in the age structure in the years to be compared. During the period 1979-92, declines are evident in all of the categories presented.

Appendix Table 5: *Live births, stillbirths, infant mortality and abortions, England, 1960-92*

Trends are discussed in this chapter.

Appendix Table 6: *Congenital malformations - trends in selected malformations, England, 1980, 1985, 1991 and 1992*

Trends are discussed in this chapter.

Appendix Table 7: *Cancer registrations, England and Wales, 1988 (males)*

The table indicates the distribution of cancer registrations in males at different ages. At all ages combined, cancers of the lung, large intestine (including rectum) and prostate account for almost half of the registrations. In childhood, a high proportion of cancers are attributable to leukaemias, lymphomas, tumours of the central nervous system, and embryonic tumours such as neuroblastomas and retinoblastomas. At older ages, cancer of the lung is the major cause registered. In the oldest age-group presented (85 years and over), prostate cancer accounts for almost as many registrations as lung cancer.

Appendix Table 8: *Cancer registrations, England and Wales, 1988 (females)*

In childhood, the pattern of female cancers is broadly similar to that in males. However, in the 25-44 years age-group cancers of the breast (35%) and cervix (17%) predominate. At older ages, breast cancer continues to account for many registrations, although cancers of the lung and large intestine also occur in substantial numbers.

Appendix Table 9: *Immunisation uptake, England, 1980-91/92*

The information presented in this table is discussed in Chapter (see page 164).

Appendix Table 10: *Cumulative total of AIDS cases by exposure category, England, to 31 December 1992*

Recent trends in AIDS cases are discussed in Chapter 6 (see page 150).

Appendix Figure 1: *Weekly deaths, England and Wales, 1991 and 1992, and expected deaths, 1992*

This figure illustrates the week-by-week registrations of deaths from all causes at ages one year and over for 1991 and 1992. These can be compared with the expected values for 1992 based on the previous 10 years.

References

1. Department of Health and Social Security. *On the State of the Public Health: the annual report of the Chief Medical Officer of the Department of Health and Social Security for the year 1987.* London: HMSO, 1988; 4, 72-82.
2. Charlton JR, Hartley RM, Silver R, Holland WW. Geographical variation in mortality from conditions amenable to medical intervention in England and Wales. *Lancet* 1983; i: 691-6.

CHAPTER 2

THE NATION'S HEALTH

(a) Public health in England

The Public Health Network

An effective public health function is essential to improve the health of the population. The strategy for health White Paper[1] stated that "the Department of Health will be exploring ways of creating national and local networks to draw together the scarce public health skills and widespread specialist knowledge to take the strategy for health forward". Ultimately, such networks will extend widely over public health issues, but building networks to encompass the full range of individuals and organisations that contribute to the public health is a long-term aim. An essential first step in this process was taken during 1992 by the creation of the Public Health Network: its role is to draw together public health skills, to facilitate communications across the whole field of public health, and to identify sources of expertise. Membership of this national Public Health Network includes the Chief Medical Officer, all 14 Regional Directors of Public Health (RDsPH), and representatives from the Office of Population Censuses and Surveys (OPCS), the Health Education Authority (HEA), the Faculty of Public Health Medicine, the Association of Directors of Public Health, the Communicable Disease Surveillance Centre (CDSC) of the Public Health Laboratory Service (PHLS) and heads of academic departments of public health medicine. Two meetings were held during 1992 to begin to explore the detailed aims and methods of working. This work will be continued in 1993, and mechanisms to ensure rapid communication will be put in place.

Surveillance of the public health function

In the summer of 1990, the Department of Health (DH) set up a surveillance programme to examine the progress made towards implementation of the Health Circular HC(88)64 *Health of the Population: responsibilities of Health Authorities*[2], and to determine the impact of the National Health Service and Community Care Act 1990[3] and the proposed strategy for health[1,4] on the public health function.

As part of this continued surveillance of the impact of reforms on the public health function, all District Directors of Public Health (DDsPH) were sent a questionnaire during 1991 by North Western Regional Health Authority's (RHA's) Department of Public Health Medicine. Provisional results were available in August 1992. Replies were received from 158 of 191 Districts, an 82% response rate. Of the responders, 96% reported that a DDPH had been appointed and 90% that he or she was an executive member of the District Health Authority (DHA). At the time of the survey only 37% were part of a commissioning/purchasing consortium. Most DDsPH were aligned with the purchasing function of the DHA and had begun to withdraw from working directly with provider units.

Health needs assessment and development of health outcome measures were both identified as key roles for Departments of Public Health Medicine. Most DDsPH identified the establishment of close links with their resident population and alliances with other agencies as central to their emerging role; a wide variety of methods had been adopted to achieve these goals.

The survey confirmed difficulties previously identified in the provision of public health medicine advice to Family Health Services Authorities (FHSAs); indeed several respondents reported that their FHSA did not receive any such advice.

This programme of surveillance of the public health function, including a follow-up to the 1991 survey, will continue during 1993.

Further development of the public health function

Although the principles outlined in the report *Public Health in England*[5] remain unchanged, the National Health Service (NHS) reforms and the impact of strategy for health have led to changes in the arrangements needed for implementation of the public health function[2]. During 1992, a small Working Group under the Chairmanship of Dr Michael Abrams, then Deputy Chief Medical Officer, was asked "to undertake a review of HC(88)64 in the light of the NHS reforms and to develop new guidance by late Spring 1993". Its remit includes the organisation of communicable disease control and the control of non-infectious environmental hazards.

Review of infectious disease control legislation

One of the recommendations in the report *Public Health in England*[5] was that DH should "revise the Public Health (Control of Disease) Act 1984 with a view to producing a more up to date and relevant legislative backing to control of communicable disease and infection". Following consultation on the options for change, work has begun towards future legislation. A series of seminars and meetings with health and local authority staff and other public health professionals continued this process of consultation and detailed policy development. DH and the Department of the Environment issued joint guidance[6] in October 1991 to remind health and local authorities of the collaborative arrangements required for communicable disease control. The need for further guidance will be considered as part of the work of the Abrams Committee.

Training in public health medicine

DH continued its support of the training posts already established since 1988 for doctors to train in the specialty of public health medicine. In addition, 34 new posts were funded, of which 8 will be based in academic departments. Following publication of the report *Public Health in England*[5], DH commissioned a survey of training needs for consultants in communicable disease control (CsCDC). Pump-priming finance of over £500,000 has since been made available from a central fund for short-term training of CsCDC. A further £164,000 were allocated to provide training for public health professionals in legal aspects of their work. In June 1992, DH funded and organised the second 2-day national conference for CsCDC and has planned a third conference for 1993.

References

1. Department of Health. *Health of the Nation: a strategy for health in England.* London: HMSO, 1992 (Cm. 1986).
2. Department of Health. *Health services management: health of the population: responsibilities of Health Authorities.* Heywood (Lancashire): Department of Health, 1988 (Health Circular: HC(88)64).
3. *National Health Service and Community Care Act 1990.* London: HMSO, 1990.
4. Department of Health. *Health of the Nation: a consultative document for health in England.* London: HMSO, 1991 (Cm. 1523).
5. *Public Health in England: The Report of the Committee of Inquiry into Future Development of the Public Health Function.* London: HMSO, 1988 (Cm. 289). Chair: Sir Donald Acheson.
6. Department of Health and Department of the Environment. *Communicable disease control.* London: Department of Health, 1991 (Executive Letter: EL(91)123).

(b) Regional perspectives

North East and North West Thames

Last year's Report highlighted issues surrounding the health of black and ethnic minority groups[1]. Between them, North East and North West Thames RHAs contain the largest and most varied ethnic population in England. According to the 1991 Census, ethnic minorities formed 16.1% of the population in North West Thames, and 13.9% in North East Thames. Accordingly, both RHAs have a specific interest in the health of ethnic minorities and continue to support the work of the Health and Ethnicity Programme across both Regions. Several initiatives on ethnic health were taken forward by this bi-Regional programme during 1992.

Dental health in ethnic minorities

South Asian and Vietnamese children, especially in the pre-school age-group, appear to have higher rates of dental caries than white children. During 1992, dental health among children in ethnic minority groups was assessed in the two North Thames Regions. A survey, carried out with the help of District dental health officers, showed that Asian 5-year-olds had poorer dental health than their white counterparts[2]. In one District, Hounslow and Spelthorne, there were also indications that Asian children's dental health had deteriorated between 1988 and 1992. However, the dental health of older Asian children was as good, if not better, than that of white children. A need for better targeting of dental services and health education for South Asian and Vietnamese mothers was identified in the report.

The health of refugees

London is the destination for 90% of all asylum seekers to Britain, and many of these make their homes in inner-city areas. A study of refugees and asylum seekers was carried out across the two Regions in 1992. The study found 79,000

51

refugees in North East Thames and 37,000 in North West Thames, as well as 254 unaccompanied refugee children across both Regions[3]. Two major factors affected their health care; refugees have poor access to health services, mainly due to a lack of interpreting services, and some health professionals do not understand the status of refugees and view them as illegal immigrants without entitlement to health care. This study has led to further research on the reception and aftercare health services provided to asylum seekers in both Regions.

Suicide in ethnic minorities

In response to anecdotal reports that suicides were frequent among refugees, the records of 559 suicides from Greater London Coroners' Courts in the two health Regions were examined, alongside an analysis of national data on mortality by country of birth for the years 1979-85. No evidence of an increase in suicide among refugees could be found, but there was an excess suicide rate among Asian women aged 15-34 years, and especially in Pakistani and Bangladeshi women aged 15-24 years. The 12 suicides among Asian women found in the Coroners' records were examined for clues as to contributory factors: most had a history of serious psychiatric disturbance, but the influence of family conflict was difficult to define. These findings emphasise a need to maintain services, such as women's refuges, which can provide adequate facilities and support for young women from ethnic minority groups.

Trent

Trent, one of the largest health Regions in England, includes South Yorkshire and parts of the East Midlands. The resident population is over 4.6 million with over 200,000 from black and ethnic minority groups (4.4% of the total). Leicestershire has a particularly large ethnic minority population, mainly of Indian origin. Last year's Report[1] highlighted differences in health between ethnic minority groups, including excess coronary heart disease (CHD) and stroke mortality in those born in the Indian Subcontinent, and excess stroke mortality in those born in the Caribbean and African Commonwealth. The Report also drew attention to the difficulties of comparative analysis due to lack of information. While some of the major health-related databases include country of birth as a data item, few include ethnicity - which is increasingly relevant as the proportions of UK-born individuals increase among ethnic minority populations. Without such information to assess the health needs of ethnic minority populations, there is a danger that health authorities and their partners in local 'healthy alliances' may not commit adequate resources to targeted health improvement programmes.

In Trent, as in other parts of the country, problems caused by lack of broad-based data have been alleviated by local research, in which the study of local evidence of health needs among ethnic minority groups has provided impetus for change. In Leicestershire, for example, blood collection in local antenatal clinics helped to define the prevalence of sickle-cell disorder and thalassaemia, and these findings gave an added urgency to the provision of screening and counselling services. In Southern Derbyshire, needs assessment work identified a high prevalence of diabetes mellitus among local Asians. In response, the health authority appointed a community dietitian, a health promotion officer and a diabetes liaison nurse to work mainly with the Asian community. Other work has highlighted the potential health hazards of surma, a lead-based eye cosmetic used on children in some Asian groups. Health visitors' observations of surma use, together with chemical analysis of locally collected samples, confirmed the hazard and led to a programme to raise awareness of the risks involved. In Rotherham, the largest single ethnic minority group have their origins in rural Pakistan: surveys indicate high levels of illiteracy in English and other languages among this group. Perinatal mortality is about three times that among the local non-Asian population, and there is evidence of high rates of CHD and diabetes mellitus. As part of their response to these challenges, Rotherham FHSA (in conjunction with other agencies) has set up a project to develop communication between this ethnic group and health and social care services and to increase awareness of this community's needs among health care workers.

Local research in several Trent Districts has also identified examples of cultural insensitivity in pre-existing services. Armed with such information, purchasers and providers can take appropriate corrective action. The Patient's Charter[4] provides a stimulus and a framework for these improvements in service to the whole of the local population.

Yorkshire

Accidents are a major cause of death, particularly among young people - as recognised by their inclusion as a key area in the strategy for health[5]. Facilities to cope with accidents, and particularly major trauma, have been extensively reviewed in recent years, and a number of studies and commissioned reports[6,7,8] have indicated that the setting up of designated major trauma centres may be the best way to ensure the most effective management of critical injuries. This issue was taken up in Yorkshire in 1990, when the Leeds School of Public Health was commissioned to investigate health service workloads in relation to patients with severe injuries caused by major trauma. The results of this study were published in 1992[9]; they were discussed by the Regional Medical Advisory Group and the conclusions were accepted as a baseline for the development of a Regional policy on major trauma. This policy was further developed in a workshop at which members of the Regional Medical Advisory Group were able to identify the key issues to be incorporated into a major trauma policy document.

It was agreed that major trauma causes significant mortality and morbidity in the Region. Reduction of the mortality and morbidity caused by major trauma will require the development of an integrated service which addresses five key aspects. First, primary prevention - which must include the development of an effective road transport policy, road planning and construction to take account of drivers' (and others') safety, effective measures to eliminate driving under the influence of alcohol, and other aspects of traffic policing and public education. Second, an effective immediate response at the site of an accident and prompt transport to hospital must be ensured by the provision of trained ambulance crews with agreed assessment approaches and a policy to ensure rapid transfer to hospital with intervention only as necessary. For the emergency care and stabilisation of patients at receiving hospitals it was agreed that there should be a system of accreditation for acute hospitals across the Region, leading to the designation of major trauma reception hospitals - which must have 24-hour availability of consultant-led teams, staffed emergency theatres and full supporting specialist services. Few hospitals would be able to have every possible specialist facility on site, but referral and transfer to tertiary specialist care - such as neurosurgery or burns units - must be ensured; further investigation of the requirement for tertiary services in the Region will be set up. Finally, follow-up and rehabilitation should not be forgotten - indeed, early access to expert and comprehensive rehabilitation services for all survivors of major trauma was regarded as a key issue.

The Yorkshire Regional policy for major trauma is being developed and further research is clearly needed. The issues identified above will provide a focus for this research and should enable the Region to enhance its provision of effective major trauma services. The role of major trauma centres is also being investigated in a study in which DH is funding a pilot major trauma centre in Stoke-on-Trent, with comparisons being made to services in Preston and Hull. Results of this evaluation should become available towards the end of 1994.

References

1. Department of Health. *On the State of the Public Health 1991: the annual Report of the Chief Medical Officer of the Department of Health for the year 1991.* London: HMSO, 1992; 54-77.
2. Regional Health and Ethnicity Programme. *Dental health and ethnic minority children.* London: North West and North East Thames Regional Health Authorities, 1992.
3. Karmi G, ed. *Refugees and the National Health Service.* London: North West and North East Thames Regional Health Authorities Health and Ethnicity Programme, 1992.
4. Department of Health. *The Patient's Charter.* London: Department of Health, 1991.
5. Department of Health. *The Health of the Nation: a strategy for health in England.* London: HMSO, 1992 (Cm. 1986).
6. Royal College of Surgeons. *Report of the Working Party on the Management of Patients with Major Injuries.* London: Royal College of Surgeons, 1988.
7. Department of Transport. *Road Accidents in Great Britain 1985.* London: HMSO, 1986.
8. British Orthopaedic Association. *The Management of Trauma in Great Britain.* London: British Orthopaedic Association, 1989.
9. Airey M, Franks A. The epidemiology of major trauma in the Yorkshire Health Region. Leeds: Leeds School of Public Health, 1992.

(c) Smoking and health

Prevalence

Whilst the prevalence of cigarette smoking among adults continues to fall[1], the rate of reduction gives no cause for complacency. The strategy for health White Paper[2] sets out to reduce the prevalence of cigarette smoking to no more than 20% by the year 2000 in men and women alike, and to reduce cigarette consumption by at least 40% from 1990 values in the same period. These challenging targets are ahead of the underlying rate of decline shown in Table 2.1. To achieve these targets, the strategy for health[2] sets out a comprehensive programme to take action on pricing, to provide health education and to ensure effective controls on advertising (see page 68). It also emphasises the key role of health authorities in leading moves to improve the health of local people, including action to reduce smoking.

Table 2.1: *Prevalence of cigarette smoking in adults (aged 16 years and over) in England, 1974-90*

Year	Men %	Women %
1974	51	40
1978	44	36
1982	37	33
1984	35	32
1986	34	31
1988	32	30
1990	31	28
2000 target	*20*	*20*

Note: This table shows prevalence for England alone, unlike previous years.

Source: OPCS

Smoking in pregnancy

In 1992, DH provided a second grant of £500,000 to the HEA to fund a project to reduce smoking in pregnancy, one of the key targets in the strategy for health[2] (see Table 2.2). It will provide information and support to encourage pregnant women, and those hoping to become pregnant, to stop smoking. A secondary aim is to ensure that they do not start smoking again after giving birth.

Table 2.2: *Percentage of pregnant women smoking before and during pregnancy in Great Britain, 1985-90*

Year	All mothers		Mothers who smoked before but gave up during pregnancy %
	Smoked before pregnancy %	Smoked during pregnancy %	
1985	39	30	24
1990	38	28	27
2000 target	-	-	*33*

Source: Infant Feeding Surveys[3]

Teenage smoking

1992 was the fourth year of the joint DH/HEA teenage smoking programme. Although remarkably high rates of awareness have been found about anti-smoking messages in the press and on television, this awareness has unfortunately not translated into behavioural change. Teenage smoking figures appear to be fairly stable (see Table 2.3)[4].

Efforts to reduce teenage smoking may need to take into account smoking prevalence among friends and relations. Most teenagers who smoke cigarettes have parents or siblings who also smoke: compared with children whose parents do not smoke, children of parents who do are themselves two-and-a-half times more likely to smoke.

Table 2.3: *Prevalence of regular* cigarette smoking in children (aged 11-15 years) in England, 1982-92*

Year	Boys %	Girls %	Total %
1982	11	11	11
1984	13	13	13
1986	7	12	10
1988	7	9	8
1990	9	11	10
1992†	9	10	10
1994 target			<6

*Regular smoking defined as usually smoking at least one cigarette per week.
†Provisional figures.

Source: OPCS

In December 1992, a campaign to extend the message of the teenage smoking programme to parents who smoke started in northern England. The campaign, which includes television advertising and a local 'healthy alliance' in West Yorkshire, aims to encourage parents to stop smoking and thereby reduce the ill-effects of passive smoking and set a good example to their children.

Passive smoking

The strategy for health[2] makes clear the Government's wish to protect non-smokers from the effects of tobacco smoke. Targets for the provision of smoke-free areas include:

- At least 80% of public places to be covered by effective non-smoking policies by 1994;

- The large majority of employees to be covered by workplace non-smoking policies by 1995; *and*

- The whole NHS to work towards a virtually smoke-free environment for staff, patients and visitors as rapidly as possible.

Guidance has been produced and widely distributed by the Department of the Environment and the Health and Safety Executive and encouraging progress has been made.

By 31 December 1992, all sales of tobacco on NHS premises were stopped, although long-stay patients who do not want to stop smoking and have no alternative source of supply are exempted from this ruling. By mid-1993, all NHS premises will be required to implement non-smoking policies to ensure that the NHS is virtually smoke-free, except for the provision of a limited number of separate smoking rooms.

Smoking cessation

The recently renegotiated general practitioner (GP) contract emphasises the need to achieve the strategy for health's smoking targets[2]. All primary health care teams are encouraged to record smoking status and to offer advice on smoking cessation. The anti-smoking charity QUIT continues to receive financial support for its project to provide GPs with the training and resources needed to manage smoking cessation within their practices.

Inter-Departmental Task Force on smoking

Action to achieve the strategy for health's targets[2] will clearly involve many Government Departments and Agencies, and several inter-Departmental Task Forces have been set up to co-ordinate these efforts. The Task Force on smoking has already begun work.

Tar yield

Adoption of an European Community (EC) Directive has led to Regulations to reduce the tar yield of cigarettes, which came into force in November 1992. Apart from transitional arrangements for cigarettes already produced, these Regulations prevent the supply of cigarettes that yield more than 15 mg of tar from 1 January 1993, and more than 12 mg of tar from 1 January 1998. From January 1992, tar and nicotine yields must be displayed on all cigarette packets.

Oral snuff

Following adoption of another EC Directive, Regulations will come into force on 1 January 1993 to ban certain types of tobacco for oral use, including oral snuff. The United Kingdom (UK) strongly supported this Directive.

References

1. Office of Population Censuses and Surveys. *General Household Survey: cigarette smoking 1972 to 1990.* London: OPCS Information Branch, 1991 (OPCS Monitor SS 91/3).
2. Department of Health. *The Health of the Nation: a strategy for health in England.* London: HMSO, 1992 (Cm. 1986).
3. White A, Freeth S, O'Brien M. *Infant Feeding 1990.* London: HMSO, 1992.
4. Office of Population Censuses and Surveys. *Smoking among secondary school children in 1990.* London: HMSO, 1991 (Social Survey Report: SS 1337).

(d) Alcohol misuse

Consumption

The consumption of alcohol in sensible quantities and in appropriate circumstances provides many people with enjoyment. But a distinction must be made between sensible drinking and excessive or inappropriate drinking.

Surveys of alcohol consumption in England and Wales during the last few years show that 27% of men and 11% of women drink more than the recommended sensible limits of 21 and 14 units of alcohol per week, respectively[1]; 6% of men and 1% of women are very heavy drinkers, consuming more than 50 units and 35 units per week, respectively[1,2]. Consumption of alcohol within the recommended sensible limits is unlikely to cause harm, but sustained drinking above these levels contributes to a wide range of health and social problems. It is also generally acknowledged that there is a broad correlation between a society's total alcohol consumption per head and alcohol-related harm; although the UK has a lower average alcohol consumption than many other European countries, the harm that does occur leaves no room for complacency.

During 1991, alcohol consumption was 8.95 litres of pure alcohol per head of the population aged 15 years and over (this figure applies to the full calendar year, as opposed to that quoted in last year's Report[3]). There has been a slight downward trend since 1989[4], which may be related to economic factors. The proportion of total alcohol consumption by beverage type shows striking changes over the last 20 years. In 1970, when total alcohol consumption per head of population was 6.88 litres, the proportions consumed were 72% beer, 17% spirits, 9% wine and 2% cider; whereas in 1992, the provisional proportions were 53% beer and lager, 22% spirits, 21% wine and 4% cider. This changing pattern of British drinking shows a striking move away from beer to spirits and especially wine.

Targets and initiatives

The strategy for health White Paper[5] sets a specific target to reduce the proportion of heavy drinkers by 30% by the year 2005 (see page 67). A large number of initiatives to achieve this target have been proposed, some of which build on a series of co-ordinated inter-Departmental initiatives that followed publication of the Lord President's Report *Action on Alcohol Misuse* in 1991[6]. Action to help to achieve this target includes:

-   health to be one of the factors taken into account by the Chancellor of the Exchequer when deciding the appropriate level of alcohol duties in any year;

-   a strengthened commitment within the framework of the family health services to promote sensible drinking;

- joint consideration within the Alcohol Trade Associations of an agreed format for the display of customer information on alcohol units at points of sale;

- a new initiative to monitor public awareness of sensible drinking limits;

- encouragement of employers to introduce, and to evaluate the impact of, workplace alcohol policies; *and*

- support for expansion and improvement of voluntary sector service provision, including allocation of £4 million over three years to Alcohol Concern, and through Alcohol and Drug specific grants to a total of £2.1 million in 1992/93.

In early 1993, DH hopes to publish a special resource pack, which will include emphasis on health promotion and treatment of alcohol problems for use by GPs and primary health care teams.

There are some encouraging signs that awareness of alcohol problems may be increasing: an evaluation of HEA's 'Drinkwise 1992' campaign indicated that 75% of the general public is becoming more aware of safe levels of drinking and the concept of units of alcohol. However, the Government recognises that concerted action between Departments and across the health services will be required if problems connected with excessive and inappropriate consumption of alcohol are to be tackled successfully.

References

1. Office of Population Censuses and Surveys. *General Household Survey*. London: OPCS Information Branch, 1991.
2. Office of Population Censuses and Surveys. *Drinking in England and Wales in the late 1980s*. London: OPCS Social Service Division, 1991.
3. Department of Health. *On the State of the Public Health: the annual report of the Chief Medical Officer of the Department of Health for the year 1991*. London: HMSO, 1992; 47.
4. Department of Health. *On the State of the Public Health: the annual report of the Chief Medical Officer of the Department of Health for the year 1989*. London: HMSO, 1990; 40.
5. Department of Health. *The Health of the Nation: a strategy for health in England*. London: HMSO, 1992 (Cm. 1986).
6. Lord President of the Council. *Lord President's report on action against alcohol misuse*. London: HMSO, 1991.

(e) Drug misuse

In England the total number of addicts notified to the Chief Medical Officer at the Home Office continued to rise at a rate similar to that in recent years. Compared with 1991[1], 1992 saw a 21% rise in first notifications to 9,700, and a 17% rise in renotifications to 15,000; the combined total of 24,700 notifications is the highest number yet recorded. The number of newly notified addicts increased in all age-groups between 1991 and 1992. Nearly three-quarters of new addicts were under 30 years old, such that the average age of new addicts in 1992 fell for the first time since 1985 to just under 27 years. The proportion of all those notified who were addicted to heroin fell from 72% in 1991 to 69% in

1992, but this is balanced by an increase in methadone use, which now accounts for over 40% of notifications. Less than 10% of notified addicts were reported to be addicted to cocaine, although this proportion has increased since 1990.

The highest notification rates continue to be found in London, Merseyside and the North West, and for the first year notifications were received from every health District in England. Before 1990, most notifications came from GPs, but in 1992 this proportion had fallen to 35%; 50% of notifications came from drug treatment centres and hospitals, and 15% from prison medical officers and police surgeons.

The proportion of those first notified who misuse drugs by injection has fallen from 65% in 1990 to 54% in 1992. There was an even larger fall in renotified injecting drug misusers, from 66% in 1990 to 53% in 1992. These changes in injection practice are important in terms of HIV risk, and probably reflect the increasing proportion of drug misusers now being treated with oral methadone.

HIV-seroprevalence among drug misusers

In England, known HIV-seropositivity among injecting drug misusers is generally low, with an estimated seroprevalence below 2% for most of England, rising to 6-13% in London. These figures compare with HIV-seroprevalence rates of 30% in Amsterdam and 30-40% in Rome and Milan.

Harm minimisation strategies

Long-term drug injectors in the UK appear to have high levels of awareness about HIV infection and AIDS. Many drug misusers have changed their drug injecting behaviour to reduce the risk of acquiring HIV infection. In the mid-1980s, well over half of all drug injectors shared needles and syringes, whereas by 1990 20% of injectors who attended a syringe exchange scheme, and 40% who did not, still shared needles and syringes[2]. Needle and syringe exchange schemes, introduced in 1987 and now numbering over 300 in England and Wales, and targeted health education will probably have contributed to this welcome trend.

However, the dangers to public health of the spread of HIV infection leave no room for complacency. The strategy for health White Paper[3] includes a specific target related to drug misuse and injecting behaviour as part of an overall objective to reduce the incidence of HIV infection (see page 71).

Volatile substance misuse

Solvent and volatile substance misuse continues to be an important addiction problem amongst young people, and shows no sign of abating. In 1991, the most recent year for which figures are available, there were 122 deaths due to volatile substance misuse and half of them were in people aged 15-19 years. An all-Party Parliamentary Group on the Prevention of Solvent and Volatile Substance Misuse was formed in 1991, with the aim of providing an effective forum to address this problem and to encourage preventive measures.

During 1992 there were two new initiatives. The Prevention Working Group of the Advisory Council on the Misuse of Drugs began to collect evidence on solvent misuse for a report to be published in 1993. DH also launched a national publicity campaign on solvent misuse: as well as television and press advertising, the booklet *Solvents - A Parent's Guide*[4] was widely distributed to raise awareness about this problem.

European Drug Prevention Week

European Drug Prevention Week was a major EC initiative held under the UK Presidency in November 1992 (see page 199). Its aim was to raise awareness of drug misuse, particularly among parents, teachers and young people. In London, a media seminar featured keynote speeches from HRH the Princess of Wales, the Secretary of State for Health, and the EC Commissioner for Social Affairs. There was also a conference for health professionals and an exhibition. Events and conferences were held across the country to attract sponsorship and to raise awareness of drug misuse in local communities.

The overall reaction to this initiative from the media, health professionals and local organisers has been very positive. Preliminary results from public opinion surveys of its impact among adults and children are encouraging.

References

1. Department of Health. *On the State of the Public Health: the annual report of the Chief Medical Officer of the Department of Health for the year 1991.* London: HMSO, 1992; 49.
2. Donoghoe MC, Stimson GV, Dolan KA. *Syringe Exchange in England: an overview.* London: Centre for Research on Drugs and Human Behaviour, 1992.
3. Department of Health. *The Health of the Nation: a strategy for health in England.* London: HMSO, 1992 (Cm. 1986).
4. Department of Health. *Solvents - A Parent's Guide.* London: Department of Health, 1992.

(f)   'Look After Your Heart'

The 'Look After Your Heart' (LAYH) programme, jointly funded by DH and the HEA, continues to be a focus for action to prevent CHD in England. Through national and local activities, LAYH provides information to the public and helps to make the most of the opportunities that exist everywhere to tackle CHD - a role emphasised by the strategy for health's targets for reduction in CHD and stroke[1].

Local projects

During the year, local projects continued to play an important part in the LAYH programme. £400,000 were allocated to continue the funding of eight long-term projects, which covered such topics as work with black and ethnic minority groups, community development and local media. Up to £10,000 were additionally available for each health Region to fund smaller projects.

Workplace programme

In response to demand, the LAYH Workplace programme now promotes the full range of HEA's activities, which includes advice on smoking, alcohol and AIDS as well as CHD prevention. The programme now covers 835 employers and over 4 million employees across the public and private sectors.

National promotional activities

Activities in 1992 included a month-long 'Enjoy Healthy Eating' campaign in September, intended to encourage people to eat more fibre-rich starchy .foods. Over five million leaflets were distributed through local health promotion units, ten of the largest food retail outlets and members of the Food Trade Association.

Heartbeat awards scheme

LAYH Heartbeat awards are awarded to catering establishments that offer healthy food choices, smoke-free areas and food hygiene training for their staff. After wide consultation, the scheme became locally based, with awards implemented by local teams of environmental health officers, dietitians and health promotion officers. However, the HEA remains closely involved with the scheme and is developing nationwide initiatives with the larger catering organisations.

Physical fitness

The promotion of physical fitness is an important part of the LAYH programme and was the theme of an 'LAYH Take Part' event held in Birmingham during June. The results of the Allied Dunbar National Fitness survey were published in June[2] and indicated that overall levels of fitness in the population were very low (see below). There will be consultation about the future development of a strategy to promote physical fitness in the light of the results of this survey and the targets of the strategy for health.

References

1. Department of Health. *The Health of the Nation: a strategy for health in England.* London: HMSO, 1992 (Cm. 1986).
2. Allied Dunbar National Fitness Survey. *A report on activity patterns and fitness levels commissioned by the Sports Council and the Health Education Authority: main findings.* London: Sports Council, 1992.

(g) Physical activity

Regular strenuous physical activity is associated with a lower incidence of CHD: but how much exercise, of what type, should be recommended for whom? It is difficult to draw up general guidelines without some knowledge of the population's exercise behaviour. Accordingly, the activity and fitness of English adults was assessed in the Allied Dunbar National Fitness Survey[1], which also investigated other aspects of health status and attitudes, practices and beliefs about exercise, and other lifestyle behaviours.

A representative sample of 6,000 adults was selected at random throughout the country. 4,300 completed a home interview, of whom 62% attended a subsequent physical appraisal at a specially equipped mobile laboratory; some elderly or infirm subjects were tested less rigorously in their homes.

The main finding was that 70% of men and 80% of women do not achieve the levels of regular physical activity likely to provide a health benefit at their age. Nevertheless, 80% of men and women of all ages believed themselves to be physically fit and thought (most of them wrongly) that they did enough exercise to keep fit, and a similar proportion expressed a strong belief in the contribution of exercise to health and fitness.

The strategy for health[2] contained an undertaking that the Government will, in consultation with others, develop detailed strategies to encourage appropriate levels of physical activity. The results of this survey indicate that there is considerable scope for improved awareness about appropriate exercise levels.

References

1. Allied Dunbar National Fitness Survey. *A report on activity patterns and fitness levels commissioned by the Sports Council and the Health Education Authority: main findings.* London: Sports Council, 1992.
2. Department of Health. *The Health of the Nation: a strategy for health in England.* London: HMSO, 1992 (Cm. 1986).

(h) Nutrition

The strategy for health

The strategy for health[1] proposed the formation of a Nutrition Task Force to help to meet the nutritional elements of the targets in the CHD and stroke key area. These include specific targets to reduce the contributions of total fat and of saturated fatty acids to food energy (by 12% and 35%, respectively), and for a substantial reduction in the prevalence of obesity; to achieve the target for reduced systolic blood pressure in the adult population will also require a lower intake of sodium (principally from common salt).

The Task Force, chaired by Professor Dame Barbara Clayton, consists of members from various industrial, academic and voluntary sectors as well as a number of Government Departments, and first met in December 1992. The Task Force will propose a plan of action and means to monitor progress towards the targets. The main work of the Task Force will be carried out by four Working Groups that will address specific areas - the food chain; catering; education (schools, public and media); and NHS issues and professional training.

Folic acid and the prevention of neural tube defects

In 1991, a Medical Research Council (MRC) study concluded that women who had already had a baby with a neural tube defect (NTD) could reduce the risk of recurrence by dietary supplementation with folic acid around the time of conception. Immediate guidance was issued by Chief Medical and Nursing Officers that women who had had a child with NTD should take 5 mg (or 4 mg if a preparation became available) of supplementary folic acid daily while they were planning to conceive and for the first 12 weeks of pregnancy[2]. The Chief Medical Officer also set up an Expert Group chaired by Professor Dame June Lloyd to consider the findings from the study and to make recommendations.

The Expert Group prepared a report[3] which was circulated with a letter of guidance from the Chief Medical and Nursing Officers[4] in December 1992. The Expert Group endorsed the earlier advice for women who had had a child with NTD, and advised that women who had not had a child with NTD (who account for 95% of all NTD births) should take a daily supplement of 0.4 mg of folic acid for the same interval, at the same time as increasing dietary folate through changes in food intake or by food fortification.

Nutrition of elderly people

During 1992, DH published the report *The Nutrition of Elderly People*[5] from the Committee on Medical Aspects of Food Policy (COMA). An Expert Group, chaired by Professor Malcolm Hodkinson, had reviewed all available information and made recommendations about the nutrition of this growing section of the population. A balanced diet and healthy eating, with regular physical activity appropriate to the general level of health, was recommended. The report emphasised that foods should be carefully chosen to ensure an adequate intake of all nutrients, especially if the amount of food consumed falls, and highlighted the risk of vitamin D deficiency among elderly people who do not go out of doors. Older or more frail elderly people seem to be most vulnerable to nutritional deficiency, especially as a result of repeated episodes of ill health, and would benefit from expert dietetic advice.

The Group made several recommendations about research where there were inadequate data. Since publication of the report, it has been agreed that a National Diet and Nutrition Survey of elderly people will be supported jointly by DH and the Ministry of Agriculture, Fisheries and Food. A year of field work to gather information will begin in September 1994.

'Infant Feeding 1990'

DH commissioned the fourth 5-yearly survey[6] of infant feeding practices. For the first time, the study included the whole of the UK. After adjusting for demographic changes between the population of 1985 and that of 1990, a small downward trend in breast-feeding was recorded. In Britain (earlier surveys did not cover Northern Ireland so trends for the whole UK cannot be assessed), 63% of babies were initially breast-fed, falling to 50% by 2 weeks-of-age and only 39% at 6 weeks-of-age. Infants were followed up to the age of 9 months, by which time all were on a mixed diet of milk and solid foods. This survey has provided important data for a recently established COMA Expert Group on Weaning and the Weaning Diet, chaired by Professor Forrester Cockburn, which is expected to report in 1993.

References

1. Department of Health. *The Health of the Nation: a strategy for health in England.* London: HMSO, 1992 (Cm. 1986).
2. Department of Health. *Folic acid in the prevention of neural tube defects.* London: Department of Health, 1991 (Professional Letter: PL/CMO(91)11, PL/CNO(91)6).
3. Department of Health. *Folic acid and the prevention of neural tube defects.* Heywood (Lancashire): Department of Health, 1992.
4. Department of Health. *Folic acid and the prevention of neural tube defects: guidelines on prevention.* London: Department of Health, 1992 (Professional Letter: PL/CMO(92)18, PL/CNO(92)12).
5. Department of Health. *The Nutrition of Elderly People.* London: HMSO, 1992 (Report on Health and Social Subjects no. 43).
6. White A, Freeth S, O'Brien M. *Infant Feeding 1990.* London: HMSO, 1992.

CHAPTER 3

THE STRATEGY FOR HEALTH

(a) The Health of the Nation White Paper

The White Paper *The Health of the Nation: a strategy for health in England*[1] was published in July 1992. It set out, for the first time, a coherent strategy to improve the health of the people of England with an emphasis on health in its widest sense rather than on health service delivery. The health strategy identifies five key areas, sets out national objectives and specific targets in each key area, and indicates the action needed to achieve these targets.

In addition to the full White Paper, which was distributed widely, a summary was circulated to all doctors, dentists, pharmacists and opticians, and over half a million copies of a 'popular' version - *The Health of the Nation and You*[2] - were distributed to members of the public who responded to an advertising campaign when the strategy was launched.

A major theme of the strategy is the formation of 'healthy alliances', in which different organisations and individuals are brought together to exchange ideas and information so that they can tackle health issues more effectively. The use of 'healthy settings' to help to achieve the targets is another theme in the strategy, which identifies seven settings where action can be taken to improve the health of the population: 'healthy' cities, schools, hospitals, workplaces, homes, prisons, and environments.

The strategy for health was widely welcomed: the World Health Organization (WHO), and many health care professionals, local authorities and voluntary organisations hailed it as an important initiative to help to improve the health of the population.

References

1. Department of Health. *The Health of the Nation: a strategy for health in England*. London: HMSO, 1992 (Cm. 1986).
2. Department of Health. *The Health of the Nation and you*. Heywood (Lancashire): Department of Health, 1992.

(b) Key areas and targets

The White Paper[1] identifies five key areas, which cover 27 national targets, and specifies the action required to meet these health targets. These key areas were selected on the basis of three criteria set out in the Green Paper, *The Health of the Nation: a consultative document for health in England*[2]. These requirements were that:

-   the area should be a major cause of premature death or avoidable ill-health;

-   effective interventions should be possible, offering scope for significant improvement in health; *and*

-   it should be possible to set objectives and targets and monitor progress towards these.

The Green Paper discussed 16 possible priority areas and many others were suggested during the wide consultation that followed its publication. The five key areas chosen as first order priorities for the strategy for health were coronary heart disease (CHD) and stroke; cancer; mental illness; HIV/AIDS and sexual health; and accidents.

(i)   Coronary heart disease and stroke

Objective: -	*To reduce the level of ill-health and death caused by CHD and stroke, and the risk factors associated with them.*

During the consultation, there was virtually unanimous agreement that the prevention of CHD and stroke should be included as a key area. CHD caused 26% of all deaths in 1991 and was the single most common cause of death in men and women alike: this mortality rate is one of the highest in the world. Stroke caused 12% of all deaths in 1991 and is a major cause of disability. CHD and stroke account for 2.5% and 6% of total National Health Service (NHS) expenditure, respectively. There is clear scope for preventing illness and death from both conditions. Moreover, reductions in the risk factors associated with these diseases - unbalanced diet, smoking, raised blood pressure, alcohol misuse and lack of physical activity - would also help to prevent many other illnesses.

Table 3.1: *Main targets for CHD and stroke*[1]

To reduce death rates for both CHD and stroke in people under 65 by at least 40% by the year 2000 *(Baseline 1990)*

To reduce the death rate for CHD in people aged 65-74 by at least 30% by the year 2000 *(Baseline 1990)*

To reduce the death rate for stroke in people aged 65-74 by at least 40% by the year 2000 *(Baseline 1990)*

[1]The 1990 baseline for all mortality targets represents an average of three years centred around 1990.

Action to achieve the targets for CHD and stroke (see Tables 3.1-3.3) will be needed both at a general level, with initiatives such as the 'Look After Your Heart' programme (see page 61) helping individuals to change their lifestyles through education and encouragement, and also at a specific level for the risk factors mentioned above. Initiatives concerning smoking, alcohol misuse, diet and nutrition, and physical activity are described more fully in Chapter 2 (see pages 54-65).

Table 3.2: *Risk factor targets: Diet and nutrition*

To reduce the average percentage of food energy derived by the population from saturated fatty acids by at least 35% by 2005 (to no more than 11% of food energy) *(Baseline 1990)*

To reduce the average percentage of food energy derived from total fat by the population by at least 12% by 2005 (to no more than about 35% of total food energy) *(Baseline 1990)*

To reduce the proportion of men and women aged 16-64 who are obese by at least 25% and 33% respectively by 2005 (to no more than 6% of men and 8% of women) *(Baseline 1986/87)*

To reduce the proportion of men drinking more than 21 units of alcohol per week and women drinking more than 14 units per week by 30% by 2005 (to 18% of men and 7% of women) *(Baseline 1990)*

Table 3.3: *Risk factor target: Blood pressure*

To reduce mean systolic blood pressure in the adult population by at least 5 mm Hg by 2005 *(Baseline to be derived from new national health survey)*

(ii) Cancers

Objectives:	-	*To reduce ill-health and death caused by breast and cervical cancer;*
	-	*To reduce ill-health and death caused by skin cancers by increasing awareness of the need to avoid excessive skin exposure to ultraviolet light;*
	-	*To reduce ill-health and death caused by lung cancer - and other conditions associated with tobacco use - by reducing smoking prevalence and tobacco consumption throughout the population.*

Cancer was chosen as one of the five key areas because it is a major cause of death and avoidable ill-health accounting for about 25% of all deaths in 1991[3]. Targets were set for four main types of cancer - lung, breast, cervix and skin - which together account for about 35% of all cancer deaths (see Table 3.4).

Lung cancer

Primary lung cancer is the most common tumour in men and one of the most common among women. It has a poor prognosis and only about 5% of patients are alive five years after the diagnosis is made[4]. At least 80% of lung cancers are associated with cigarette smoking. Clearly, primary prevention by action to reduce smoking prevalence must be the main way to reduce the morbidity and mortality caused by lung cancer. Therefore, as well as setting an overall target for the reduction of lung cancer, challenging targets were also set for reducing smoking prevalence among adults, pregnant women and teenagers. To achieve these targets (see Table 3.5), it will be necessary to reduce both the number of people who smoke cigarettes and the number of people who start to smoke. Both aspects are important, and focus on prevention alone is unlikely to achieve the reductions required. The targets for different population groups may also be inter-dependent: as noted in last year's Report[5], "a more marked reduction in adult smoking may be required before teenagers' attitudes are significantly affected". Some of the many initiatives set up to achieve these targets for reduction of cigarette smoking are described more fully in Chapter 2 (see page 54).

Table 3.4: *Main targets for cancers*[1]

To reduce the death rate for breast cancer in the population invited for screening by at least 25% by the year 2000 *(Baseline 1990)*

To reduce the incidence of invasive cervical cancer by at least 20% by the year 2000 *(Baseline 1986)*

To reduce the death rate for lung cancer under the age of 75 by at least 30% in men and by at least 15% in women by 2010 *(Baseline 1990)*

To halt the year-on-year increase in the incidence of skin cancer by 2005

---

[1]The 1990 baseline for all mortality targets represents an average of three years centred around 1990.

Table 3.5: *Risk factor targets: Smoking*

To reduce the prevalence of cigarette smoking to no more than 20% by the year 2000 in both men and women (a reduction of a third) *(Baseline 1990)*

To reduce consumption of cigarettes by at least 40% by the year 2000 *(Baseline 1990)*

In addition to the overall reduction in prevalence, at least 33% of women smokers to stop smoking at the start of their pregnancy by the year 2000

To reduce smoking prevalence of 11-15-year-olds by at least 33% by 1994 (to less than 6%) *(Baseline 1988)*

Breast cancer

One woman in 14 is likely to develop breast cancer at some time, and more women die from it than from any other form of cancer[3]. The goal is to save 1,250 lives each year, and has been made possible by the nationwide breast cancer screening programme for women aged 50-64 years. With early detection vital, it is good news that over 70% of women have accepted their invitation for screening (from analysis of returns on Form KC62). The priorities for this area are to maintain the high standards already achieved by the programme, and to encourage all women to take up screening invitations.

Cervical cancer

Cervical cancer is the only cancer that usually has a long pre-invasive phase and can generally be detected by examination of cells scraped easily from the surface of the cervix. In 1988, a national cervical screening programme based on computerised call-and-recall systems was introduced. Health authorities are required to invite women aged 20-64 years for cervical screening, and to recall them at least every five years. A target has been set for a 20% reduction in the incidence of cervical cancer by the year 2000. However, the slow and variable development of this cancer means that the full potential of this call-and-recall cytology programme cannot be realised until after the year 2000 (see also page 126). Priorities are to continue the development of good practice in the operation of the screening programme, and to encourage women to be screened.

Skin cancer

Skin cancer incidence has risen sharply in the last decade (see page 173). Prevention is feasible because the cause - exposure to ultraviolet radiation - is known and avoidable. One of the targets in the strategy for health is to halt the year-on-year rise in the incidence of skin cancers by 2005. To do so, the Department of Health (DH) will work with the Health Education Authority (HEA) and other allies to increase general public awareness of the harmful effects of ultraviolet irradiation and to inform susceptible individuals about how to reduce their risk.

(iii) Mental illness

Objective:	-	*To reduce ill-health and death caused by mental illness.*

Mental illness is as common as heart disease and three times as common as cancer; six million people suffer from it in the course of a year. It was selected as a key area because it affects so many people; because there is much which can and should be achieved, particularly in relation to improvements in services to reduce the harm that mental illness can cause; and because of unanimous support for its inclusion during the consultation process. Targets are shown in Table 3.6.

Table 3.6: *Main targets for mental illness*[1]

To improve significantly the health and social functioning of mentally ill people

To reduce the overall suicide rate by at least 15% by the year 2000 *(Baseline 1990)*

To reduce the suicide rate of severely mentally ill people by at least 33% by the year 2000 *(Baseline 1990)*

[1] The 1990 baseline for all mortality targets represents an average of three years centred around 1990.

The White Paper[1] identifies three broad areas for action. The first is to tackle the lack of information on the prevalence and outcomes of mental illness, so that more precise, quantifiable targets for mental health gain can be set. DH commissioned a national survey, to start in 1993 and to be completed by 1995, into the prevalence of psychiatric morbidity and the extent of social disabilities associated with mental illness: the Office of Population Censuses and Surveys (OPCS) has completed a pilot study based in five centres. Work has also been commissioned through the Research Unit of the Royal College of Psychiatrists, in co-operation with other professional groups, to establish brief standardised assessment procedures to measure symptom state, social disability and quality of life.

The second area for action is to develop a comprehensive system of psychiatric services. The Mental Health Task Force, under the leadership of Mr David King, was set up in 1992 to oversee completion of the transfer of most mental health services from obsolete asylums to a balanced range of locally based services[6]. The work of this Task Force will be fundamental to the achievement of targets for mental health. It is also essential to develop effective information systems to plan and monitor mental health services, and mechanisms for jointly purchasing such services to ensure continuity of service delivery based on an agreed strategic framework.

The further development of good practice in both primary and secondary care was identified as the final area for action. Primary health care teams are encouraged to develop, with training where appropriate, their ability to recognise, assess and manage depression, severe anxiety and suicide risk. In addition, health authorities have been urged to introduce local multidisciplinary audit of suicides and to improve supervisory and support systems for people with mental illness in the community. Many factors influence psychological health, including family life, education, housing and employment: to encourage good practice in promoting mental health at work, DH ran a stand and held a Ministerial breakfast at the Confederation of British Industry's Annual Conference in November.

(iv) HIV/AIDS and sexual health

Objectives:	-	To reduce the incidence of HIV infection;
	-	To reduce the incidence of other sexually transmitted diseases (STDs);
	-	To develop further and strengthen monitoring and surveillance;
	-	To provide effective services for diagnosis and treatment of HIV and other STDs;
	-	To reduce the number of unwanted pregnancies;
	-	To ensure the provision of effective family planning services for those people who want them.

This topic was chosen as a key area because it encompasses HIV infection and AIDS, one of the greatest challenges to public health that has arisen this century.

The related areas of sexual health and family planning are also very important to the health and well-being of individuals and families. Targets are shown in Tables 3.7 and 3.8.

Table 3.7: *Main targets for HIV/AIDS and sexual health*

To reduce the incidence of gonorrhoea by at least 20% by 1995 *(Baseline 1990)*, as an indicator of HIV/AIDS trends

To reduce by at least 50% the rate of conceptions amongst the under 16s by the year 2000 *(Baseline 1989)*

Table 3.8: *Risk factor target: HIV/AIDS*

To reduce the percentage of injecting drug misusers who report sharing injecting equipment in the previous 4 weeks from 20% in 1990 to no more than 10% by 1997 and no more than 5% by the year 2000

The White Paper[1] identifies a range of strategic objectives and individual targets. The aim is to prevent the undesired consequences of sexual activity and drug misuse - such as sexually transmitted diseases (STDs), including HIV - and to provide effective and adequate services for those who may require such facilities.

In this country, HIV is primarily transmitted through unprotected sexual intercourse (see page 150). Particular efforts must therefore be made to encourage the adoption of safer patterns of sexual behaviour, especially among succeeding generations of young people as they come to maturity, and to urge those who may already be at increased risk to modify their lifestyles or behaviour so as to reduce or to eliminate such risk. Both tasks require sustained commitment and enthusiastic, imaginative ideas.

Safer patterns of sexual behaviour in response to the HIV/AIDS pandemic should also reduce the numbers of other STDs. The long-term effects of infections such as gonorrhoea and chlamydia can often be overlooked, but infertility and ectopic pregnancies may have serious consequences for personal health. Improved education about STDs and greater access to services for their diagnosis and treatment are therefore two key ways in which health can be protected.

Ready access to information is equally important in avoiding unplanned pregnancies. Almost half of all conceptions may in some sense be unintended. By no means all such conceptions result in unwanted babies, but it seems reasonable to assume that most (if not all) pregnancies in girls under 16 years-of-age are not wanted. Young people in particular need improved access to information and education about contraception and family planning services.

The same need holds true for drug misuse, which remains a serious problem for many local communities. Sharing equipment to inject drugs is also an efficient route of transmission for HIV, and it is thus all the more important that appropriate action is taken to discourage people from engaging in such risky behaviour. There is a need for a comprehensive range of services which offers access to advice on safer drug use and safer sexual behaviour, in which particular attention should be given to the needs of those who are not usually in touch with health services.

These problems have been recognised for some years: much has already been achieved and further progress towards all the objectives was made during 1992. More detailed information is given elsewhere in this Report on HIV/AIDS (see page 150), on family planning (see page 125), and on drug misuse (see page 59). *First Steps for the NHS*[7] included a range of possible actions related to HIV/AIDS and sexual health on which the NHS can draw when developing local services.

(v) Accidents

Objective:	-	To reduce ill-health, disability and death caused by accidents.

The prevention of accidents was identified as a key area; because accidents are an important cause of injury, disability and death, particularly in young and elderly people, and can very often be avoided. The specific targets (see Table 3.9) are set for reduction in mortality because there are few good indicators of morbidity from accidents: better measures of morbidity are being developed.

Table 3.9: *Main targets for accidents*[1]

To reduce the death rate for accidents among children aged under 15 by at least 33% by 2005 *(Baseline 1990)*

To reduce the death rate for accidents among young people aged 15-24 by at least 25% by 2005 *(Baseline 1990)*

To reduce the death rate for accidents among people aged 65 and over by at least 33% by 2005 *(Baseline 1990)*

[1]The 1990 baseline for all mortality targets represents an average of the three years centred around 1990.

Many other agencies are involved in this key area; several of them have considerable experience and achievements to their names. For much of the health sector accident prevention is a new topic; nowhere is the need for healthy alliances better demonstrated. Considerable progress was made in 1992. A Task Force was established with terms of reference that include co-ordination of accident prevention research and evaluation. Eleven Government Departments, local authorities, voluntary organisations, the health service, the emergency services, industry and the media are represented.

The Royal Society for the Prevention of Accidents was awarded a grant from the special allocation of Section 64 funds for voluntary agencies announced in the

White Paper. Working closely with DH, it started a project to examine ways to develop the health service role in accident prevention. An exploratory study on accident risk and prevention in people from black and ethnic minority groups was also concluded during the year.

References

1. Department of Health. *The Health of the Nation: a strategy for health in England.* London: HMSO, 1992 (Cm. 1986).
2. Department of Health. *The Health of the Nation: a consultative document for health in England.* London: HMSO, 1991 (Cm. 1523).
3. Office of Population Censuses and Surveys. *Deaths by cause: 1991 registrations.* London: Government Statistical Service, 1992 (OPCS Monitor; DH 292/2).
4. Office of Population Censuses and Surveys. *Cancer and Survival: 1981 registrations.* London: Government Statistical Service, 1988 (OPCS Monitor; MB 88/1).
5. Department of Health. *On the State of the Public Health: the annual report of the Chief Medical Officer of the Department of Health for the year 1991.* London: HMSO, 1992; 46.
6. Department of Health. *New task force to oversee mental health services.* London: Department of Health, 1992 (Press release: H92/87).
7. NHS Management Executive. *First Steps for the NHS: recommendations of the Health of the Nation focus groups.* London: Department of Health, 1992.

(c) Second order priorities

The five key areas represent the first order priorities of the strategy for health. Many other possible areas were discussed in the consultation exercise which followed publication of the Green Paper[1]. Some areas suggested - such as maternal and child health, food safety, oral health and childhood immunisation - were felt to be sufficiently well covered by existing initiatives not to require the status of a key area, but emphasis on sustaining and building on progress already made. Other topics - such as rehabilitation, health of elderly people, asthma, back pain and drug misuse - were identified as strong candidates for future key area status, but further development and research were needed before national targets could be set.

Diabetes mellitus, hospital-acquired infection and breast-feeding were discussed in the Green Paper[1] but were not selected as key areas. They are, nevertheless, important and are not being ignored. The Clinical Standards Advisory Group (CSAG) has been asked to advise on the standard of clinical care for people with diabetes, and guidelines are being developed to achieve the targets for improvement of the care and quality of life for people with diabetes set out in the 1989 St Vincent Declaration[2] (see page 119). The CSAG has also been asked to start preliminary work on hospital-acquired infection so that it can provide further advice on this subject. The Government has set up a new National Breast-feeding Working Group to co-ordinate a programme to promote and to facilitate breast-feeding.

References

1. Department of Health. *The Health of the Nation: a consultative document for health in England.* London: HMSO, 1991 (Cm. 1523).
2. Diabetes Mellitus in Europe: a problem at all ages in all countries: a model for prevention and self care: a meeting organised by WHO and IDF Europe: proceedings. *Giornale Italiano di Diabetologia* 1990; **10** (Suppl).

(d) Implementation

The publication of the health strategy White Paper[1] is only the start of this major initiative. It is essential that the actions outlined within it are effectively implemented by the wide range of organisations involved. At a national level, the Government is committed to ensuring that everyone works together to achieve the improvement in the nation's health. Implementation of the strategy for health can be divided into five main areas.

(i) Co-ordination and development

The *Health of the Nation* initiative[1] involves many agencies and Departments and is overseen by a new Ministerial Cabinet Committee on the Health Strategy, which is chaired by the Lord President of the Council and includes Ministers from 11 Government Departments. This Cabinet Committee will co-ordinate the implementation, monitoring and development of the strategy for health in England and is responsible for effective co-ordination of issues that affect health across the United Kingdom (UK).

The three Working Groups set up to help develop the strategy for health are now assisting its implementation. These are:

- A Ministerially chaired Wider Health Working Group, which is to produce guidance on healthy alliances and health promotion in the workplace (on which reports are expected during 1993), and will consider the wider issues that may affect health;

- The Chief Medical Officer's Health of the Nation Working Group, which monitors and reviews progress towards the achievement of health targets, considers more general epidemiological and public health issues that may affect or be affected by the strategy for health, and advises on identification of possible new key areas and targets; *and*

- The Chief Executive's Working Group on NHS Implementation, which developed *First Steps for the NHS*[2], commissioned the HEA to produce *Health at Work in the NHS*[3] and is preparing *Health of the Nation Handbooks* on the five key areas for publication early in 1993 as part of its remit to oversee implementation and monitoring of the strategy's progress within the NHS. This Working Group will ensure that the White Paper's priorities are reflected in purchaser/provider plans approved by health authorities and will review the implementation plans produced by each Regional Health Authority.

(ii) Promulgation

A main priority is to ensure the continued and widespread promulgation of the strategy for health. This is taking place in a number of ways:

- *Supporting material* - demand for the summary and popular versions of the White Paper continues to be high. A cassette has been produced for blind and partially sighted people and versions for people from black and ethnic minority groups, with a supporting advertising campaign, will be launched in 1993.

- *Newsletter* - a quarterly newsletter, *Target*, was issued for the first time in December 1992 and has been widely circulated within and outside the NHS. It provides a forum for exchange of ideas and initiatives that will help to take forward work on the strategy for health.

- *Other publications* - during the latter part of 1992, several other documents related to the *Health of the Nation* initiative were published. These included *First Steps for the NHS*[2], which outlines a range of possible actions for each tier of the health service to take in 1993/94; *Health at Work in the NHS*[3], which outlines ways to ensure a safer working environment in the NHS; and *Specification of National Indicators*[4], which sets out key information that will form the basis of monitoring progress towards the achievement of national targets.

- *Conferences* - these will be held early in 1993 in each of the 14 health Regions. Representatives from all sectors interested in health will be able to meet and share ideas to take forward the strategy for health.

(iii) Implementation and development outside the NHS

The important influence of sectors outside the NHS is a central theme of the strategy for health. The White Paper includes commitments to:

- prepare guidance on policy appraisal and health;

- support voluntary organisations in taking forward work on the health targets;

- provide financial support for the UK 'Health for All Network' to establish a database for dissemination of good practice, developments and projects likely to promote 'healthy alliances';

- produce guidance on healthy workplaces;

- discuss with health professionals the development of standards of good practice and clinical guidelines and to encourage further emphasis on training in disease prevention and health promotion; *and*

- make preparations to enter the WHO 'Healthy Schools Network' in 1993.

(iv) Implementation and development inside the NHS

The NHS, as the main provider of health advice, treatment, care and support, has a central role in the implementation of the strategy for health. Among the principal activities under way, or planned, to fulfil this function are:

- incorporation of the need for health improvement into annual planning and priorities guidance;

- consideration of the setting up of task forces to stimulate and promote local action;

- appointment of Regional co-ordinators to provide strong local leadership for strategy for health initiatives;

- co-ordination of the formation of 'healthy alliances' below national level; *and*

- commitment to becoming a 'healthy employer'.

(v) Monitoring, research and reviewing

Any strategy to improve public health depends greatly on accurate data about the state of the population's health, and the early identification of changes and trends. A large number of measures are now or will shortly be in place to monitor, develop and review the strategy for health.

Monitoring

Information and indicators needed to monitor progress are being identified. The first step at national level was the publication of *Specification of National Indicators*[4], which gave full background information on the White Paper targets. A series of epidemiological overviews began with the publication of *Health of the Elderly*[5]; similar reviews on asthma, CHD and stroke will follow. An expansion of the Health Survey was announced in the White Paper[1] (see page 108): the report of the 1991 Health Survey is expected in Summer 1993. A Central Health Monitoring Unit has been set up to co-ordinate health data at a national level.

Research

Research is essential to any strategy to improve public health. DH's research and development strategy now reflects the strategy for health and will also explore areas where further work is needed to allow targets to be set (eg for rehabilitation, care of elderly people and back pain). A Concordat between the Medical Research Council and the four UK Health Departments will help to co-ordinate funding of the research needed to allow the strategy to develop.

Reviewing

For the strategy for health to be successful, it must undergo regular reviews to allow assessment and re-assessment of priorities. It is intended to produce a report of progress and plans in the Autumn of 1993.

References

1. Department of Health. *The Health of the Nation: a strategy for health in England.* London: HMSO, 1992 (Cm. 1986).
2. NHS Management Executive. *First steps for the NHS: recommendations of the Health of the Nation focus groups.* London: Department of Health, 1992.
3. Health Education Authority/NHS Management Executive. *Health at Work in the NHS.* London: Health Education Authority, 1992.
4. Department of Health. *Specification of National Indicators.* London: Department of Health, 1992.
5. Department of Health. *The Health of Elderly People: an epidemiological overview; volume I.* London: HMSO, 1992.

(e)   The way ahead

The strategy for health represents a major advance towards improved health for the people of England. At its heart is the setting out, for the first time, of priority health targets at which the nation as a whole should aim, together with action to focus effort on these target areas.

The enthusiasm generated by publication of the White Paper must be maintained. At a national level, the commitment of Ministers and senior Government officials is shown by their frequent references to the strategy, and by their attendance at conferences to promote its aims. At a local level, Regional co-ordinators must ensure a similar commitment to, and enthusiasm for, the establishment of healthy alliances. It is hoped that the publication in early 1993 of handbooks about each of the five key areas, which will contain practical information and illustrate examples of local good practice, will help to maintain the momentum of this major initiative.

CHAPTER 4

HEALTH OF MEN

Introduction

Recent Reports have looked in detail at the health of different sections of the population, such as children[1], women of reproductive age and the menopause[2], people in later life[3] and black and ethnic minorities[4]. This chapter analyses the health of adult men of approximately 18-64 years-of-age, although this age range is not applied rigidly because of variations in data availability and the importance of health determinants at younger ages.

Although life expectancy is increasing, there is a need to ensure that the additional years of life are healthy and active; health and lifestyle up to the age of 65 years are likely to be major determinants of the quality of life after that age. Men in the age-group under review are also particularly associated with the nation's economic activity and often have family responsibilities.

In 1991 there were 15,432,000 men aged 16-64 years in England, representing nearly two-thirds of the male population. The size of this group of the population has grown since 1981, most strikingly among men aged 30-44 years (up by 10.2%). The Government Actuary's 1991-based projections indicate that a fall of 13.5% will be seen in the 15-29 years age-group by 2001, but the population of men at older ages will continue to rise.

The health profiles of men and women clearly differ. More male than female births occur: a ratio of about 106 male for every 100 female births was reasonably constant for about 40 years until the 1980s, when the ratio fell to 105:100[5]. However, males have a consistently higher mortality. Fetal mortality is higher in males during early and late stages of fetal development[6], the infant mortality rate is about 20% higher in boys than girls, and higher death rates occur in males for each age-group thereafter. Based on English mortality data for 1991, an 18-year-old man has an 80% chance of survival to 65 years-of-age - much lower than an 18-year-old woman's 88% chance. Greater knowledge about the reasons for sex differences in susceptibility to common diseases might give a better understanding of disease mechanisms, to the benefit of men and women alike.

References

1. Department of Health. *On the State of the Public Health: the annual report of the Chief Medical Officer of the Department of Health for the year 1988.* London: HMSO, 1989; 65.
2. Department of Health. *On the State of the Public Health: the annual report of the Chief Medical Officer of the Department of Health for the year 1989.* London: HMSO, 1990; 54.
3. Department of Health. *On the State of the Public Health: the annual report of the Chief Medical Officer of the Department of Health for the year 1990.* London: HMSO, 1991; 68.
4. Department of Health. *On the State of the Public Health: the annual report of the Chief Medical Officer of the Department of Health for the year 1991.* London: HMSO, 1992; 54.
5. Shaw C. The sex ratio at birth in England and Wales. *Population Trends* 1989; **57:** 26-9.

6.   Waldron I. What do we know about causes of sex differences in mortality? A review of the literature. *UN Population Bull* 1986; **18**: 59-76.

(a) Mortality

Life expectancy in men is lower than that in women. Figure 4.1 shows that this difference has been seen through most of this century, although expectation of life at birth has increased substantially for men and women alike. Figure 4.2 illustrates the higher mortality rates seen in males at all ages. The relative excess in male mortality is greatest in young adults, mainly attributable to higher death rates from accidents and suicides. In 1972 a second, although smaller, peak was seen at the age of about 65 years, mainly attributable to the higher mortality rates from coronary heart disease (CHD) and lung cancer in men. Subsequent changes in mortality trends have led to a slight reduction in the male/female ratio for CHD and a striking fall for lung cancer (in 1972, the death rate for lung cancer in men aged 60-64 years was over five times that among women of the same age; in 1992, it was twice as high among men). However, in young adulthood the excess mortality in men has risen between 1972 and 1992 and the peak is broader - with substantially higher mortality among men than women between the ages of 15 and 29 years. This change is attributable, at least in part, to increases during the 1980s in deaths from suicide and AIDS among young men[1].

Figure 4.1: *Expectation of life at birth, England, 1910-12 to 1980-82*

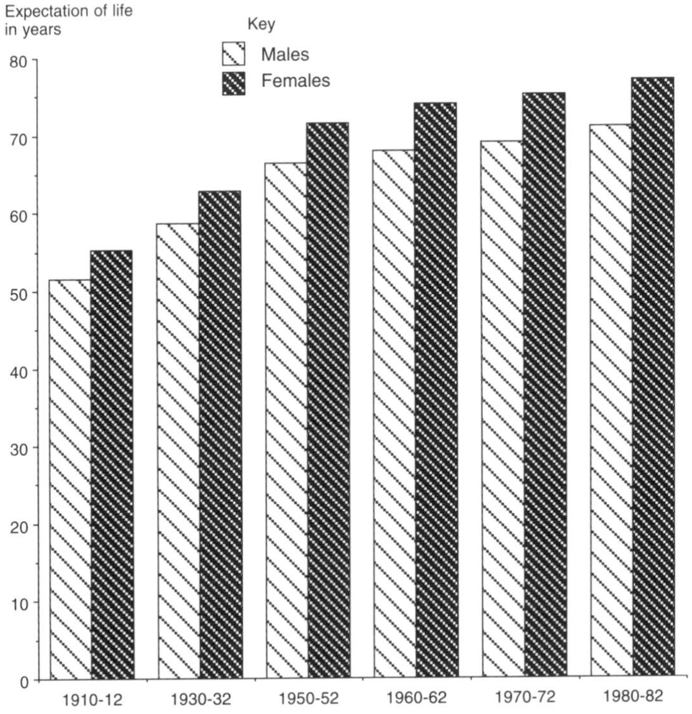

Source: Government Actuary's Department

Figure 4.2: *Sex mortality ratio* (deaths from all causes), England, 1972, 1982 and 1992*

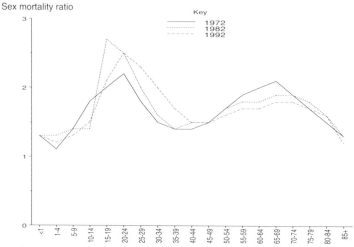

*Sex mortality ratio = male death rates/female death rates.

Source: OPCS (ICD 001-999)

What is the scope for improving these figures for male mortality? Figure 4.3 compares figures for life expectancy at birth for developed countries from the European Community (EC) and elsewhere. The United Kingdom (UK) ranks somewhere in the middle of these charts for males and females alike, which suggests substantial scope for improvements. Nevertheless, a female/male differential in life expectancy at birth is a striking feature which seems common to all these countries, and represents some 10% extra life expectancy for women.

The main causes of death in England among men and women aged 15-64 years are shown in Table 4.1. Overall, deaths from circulatory diseases predominate but, when the pattern of mortality is reviewed in different age-groups, external causes of injury and poisoning - mainly accidents and suicide - are particularly important in men below the age of 45 years (see Figure 4.4).

Table 4.1: *Selected causes of death in men and women aged 15-64 years, England, 1992*

Condition	Number of deaths	
	Men	Women
Diseases of the circulatory system	21209	7940
Coronary heart disease	*16043*	*4460*
Stroke	*2621*	*2025*
Other circulatory diseases	*2545*	*1455*
All external causes of injury and poisoning	7182	2240
Accidents and adverse effects	*3634*	*1109*
Suicide and undetermined injury	*3413*	*1046*
Other external causes	*135*	*85*
Malignant neoplasms	17282	16512
Other	9292	6305
All causes	54965	32997

81

Figure 4.3: *Expectation of life at birth, by sex and country, 1989**

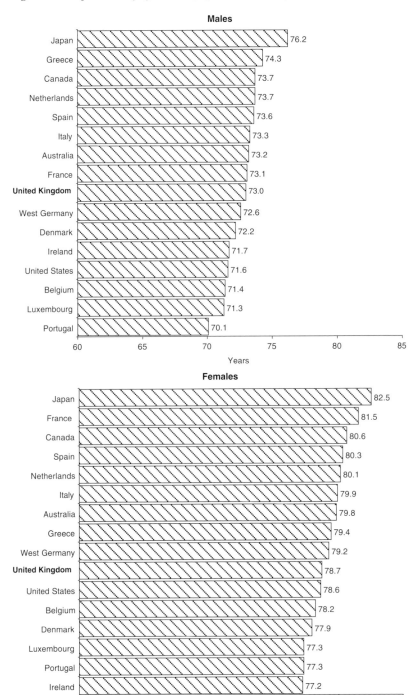

*Data for 1989 except for: Japan, UK, Denmark and Portugal 1990; Italy, Australia and USA 1988; Spain 1987; and Belgium 1986.

Source: WHO Annual of Statistics 1991

In middle age, cancers are a major cause of death, and account for about one-third of the mortality among men aged 45-64 years. Lung cancer is the leading cause of cancer mortality at these ages, as in later life, and causes one in three cancer deaths. The major gastro-intestinal cancers (oesophagus, stomach, pancreas, colon and rectum) together account for a further 28% of deaths from cancer. Many cancers can now be treated successfully and cancer registration data give a better indication of cancer occurrence than mortality data: skin cancers account for a high proportion of cancers in people at younger ages, and although testicular cancer is the most common new cancer among 25-34-year-old men, the efficacy of current treatment means that it causes only about 30 deaths annually.

Figure 4.4: *Selected causes of male deaths by age and condition, England, 1992*

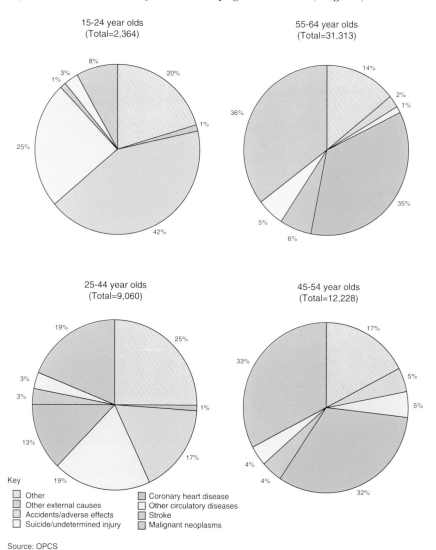

Source: OPCS

Figure 4.5: *Major causes of deaths in males aged under 65 years, European Community**

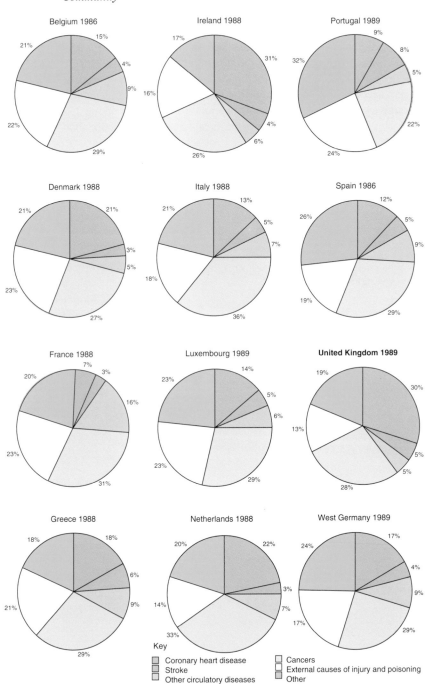

Key

☐ Coronary heart disease   ☐ Cancers
☐ Stroke   ☐ External causes of injury and poisoning
☐ Other circulatory diseases   ☐ Other

*European age-standardised death rates per 100,000 population.

Note: Percentages may not add up to 100 due to rounding.

Source: WHO HFA Indicators

Trends in mortality in men aged 15-44 years have been reviewed in recent Reports[2,3] because they have not shown the general fall in mortality seen in other age-groups in the last five to six years. Instead, mortality in this group seems to have levelled off or risen since the mid-1980s, even after demographic changes are taken into account. The Office of Population Censuses and Surveys (OPCS) has reviewed these trends in detail and largely attributes them to rises in deaths from AIDS and suicide (and "open" verdicts in Coroners' Courts). In last year's Report[3], important rises in deaths related to alcohol and drugs were also described for this age-group.

Again, international comparisons may provide a useful indication of potentially achievable improvements in these mortality figures. Major causes of death are similar in all EC countries (see Figure 4.5): circulatory diseases, cancers and external injuries and poisoning account for about 80% of deaths in UK men under 65 years-of-age and about 70-80% in other EC countries. Figure 4.6 ranks EC countries for all causes of death combined, and separately for the three major causes of death: the UK has a particularly high rate for circulatory diseases.

Figure 4.6: *Death rates from all causes and selected causes for men aged under 65 years, by country, 1988**

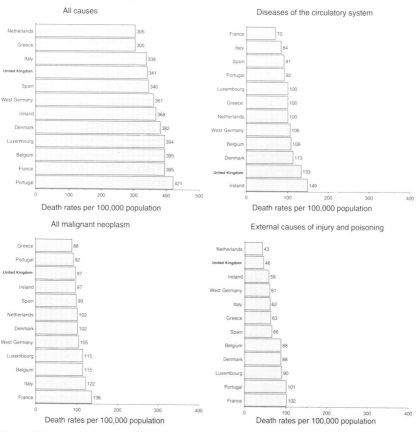

*Data for 1988 except for UK, West Germany, Portugal and Luxembourg 1989; Spain and Belgium 1986.

Source: WHO HFA indicators

85

References

1. Dunnell K. Deaths among 15-44 year olds. *Population Trends* 1991; **64**: 38-43.
2. Department of Health. *On the State of the Public Health: the annual report of the Chief Medical Officer of the Department of Health for the year 1988.* London: HMSO, 1989.
3. Department of Health. *On the State of the Public Health. the annual report of the Chief Medical Officer of the Department of Health for the year 1991.* London: HMSO, 1992; 26.

(b) Morbidity

Health means much more than the absence of death, and mortality data alone cannot be used as a reliable guide to the health of men; assessment of morbidity data provides a different, and potentially more useful, means to identify key health problems. Various sources of information exist, but each has limitations: hospital and general practitioner (GP) consultation statistics describe contacts with health services; responses to the General Household Survey (GHS) represent self-reported assessments of morbidity; and sickness absences in social security statistics relate only to the working population. Health surveys can be a useful source of information if objective measures of health are included, but national data have until recently been sparse. In general, however, available data indicate lower GP consultation rates among men than women for most illnesses, but higher rates of hospital admissions for diseases such as CHD and stroke; the overall hospital admission rate is marginally higher among men than women aged 45-64 years. Hospital admissions are a widely accepted indicator of serious health problems (see Table 4.2). For men aged 15-44 years there is a high rate of injury and poisoning, with digestive, musculoskeletal and respiratory ailments, and mental disorders also accounting for a substantial proportion of hospital admissions. At older ages (45-64 years), the overall admission rate rises and circulatory diseases and cancers become increasingly important.

Table 4.2: *Diagnosis on completion of hospital episode* per 10,000 men, England, 1989/90*

Diagnostic group	Age	
	15-44 years	45-64 years
Circulatory disease (all)	36	293
Coronary heart disease	*9*	*148*
Stroke	*3*	*27*
Other	*24*	*118*
Digestive system	122	215
Malignant neoplasm (all)	25	173
Lung cancer	*1*	*32*
Signs, symptoms and ill-defined conditions	66	140
Musculoskeletal	75	117
Injury and poisoning	179	92
Respiratory diseases	52	86
Mental disorders	63	51
All diseases and conditions	858	1533

* Finished consultant episodes (ordinary admissions and day cases).

Source: Hospital Episode Statistics, SD2A, DH

Figure 4.7: *Average episode* rates for GP consultations by sex, age and condition, England and Wales, 1981-82*

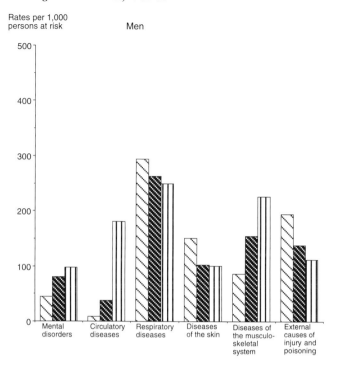

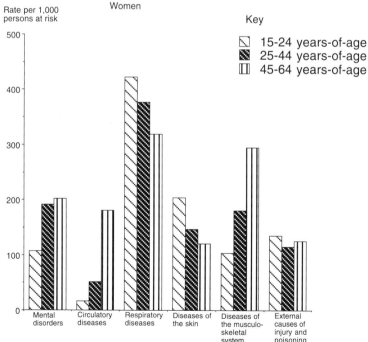

*An episode = an instance or period of sickness during which there was one or more consultations.

Source: OPCS Morbidity Statistics from General Practice 1981/82

Apart from relatively few consultations for cancer, GP consultation statistics (Table 4.3) reveal a broadly similar pattern, although in contrast to the hospital admission rates the importance of mental disorders increases among older men. Women have higher rates of GP consultations than men for most illnesses, as shown in Figure 4.7.

The GHS is a population-based survey and provides a representative picture of self-reported health trends and their variation by age and sex (see Table 4.4). A large minority of the population report the presence of a long-standing illness, disability or infirmity and about one-quarter of men (and women) aged 45-64 years report a problem of sufficient severity to limit their activity. Males report lower rates of restricted activity over the preceding 14 days due to illness or injury, and fewer consultations with a GP over the previous fortnight. Similarly, men report shorter periods of restricted activity and fewer GP consultations over the preceding year. More detailed data on the causes of long-standing illness[1] tend to confirm the patterns described from other sources.

Table 4.3: *GP consultation rates per 1,000 men, England and Wales, 1981/82*

Disease or condition	Age	
	25-44 years	45-64 years
All diseases and conditions	1984.2	3047.1
Infections and parasitic	118.6	79.8
Neoplasms	10.5	64.6
Endocrine/metabolic	31.7	97.3
Blood	2.2	9.4
Mental	173.3	227.2
Nervous system	151.2	206.2
Circulatory system	82.7	552.5
Respiratory system	339.5	393.8
Digestive system	116.3	179.7
Genito-urinary system	37.3	62.9
Skin	145.8	155.5
Musculoskeletal	253.4	435.5
Symptoms, signs	157.9	212.7
Accidents	204.5	178.6
Others	157.7	189.1

Source: OPCS, Morbidity Statistics from General Practice 1981/82 MB5 no. 1

Social security statistics of absences from work due to sickness must be interpreted with caution because of their restriction to the working population and their focus on long-term absence (short-term absences are covered by Statutory Sick Pay, and are excluded from these statistics). Nevertheless, the figures are compatible with data from other sources; most working days are lost because of musculoskeletal, circulatory, respiratory or mental disorders (see Figure 4.8).

Table 4.4: *Self-reported health data by age and sex, England, 1991*

| | 16-44 years | | 45-64 years | |
Reported condition	Men	Women	Men	Women
Long-standing illness	23	23	42	41
Limiting long-standing illness	10	11	25	25
Restricted activity due to illness or injury	9	12	12	13
Consulted GP in previous 14 days	9	17	11	17
Acute sickness: average number of restricted activity days per person per year*	18	23	31	38
Average number of NHS GP consultations per person per year*	3	6	5	6

* Based on 1990 data.

Source: GHS 1991

Reference

1.   Office of Population Censuses and Surveys. *General Household Survey 1989.* London: HMSO, 1991 (Series GHS; no. 20).

Figure 4.8: *Days of certified incapacity due to sickness and invalidity for males by cause, Great Britain, 1990/91*

Total = 356 million

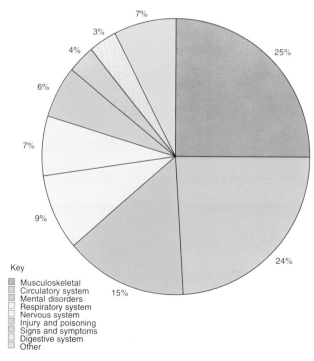

Key
- Musculoskeletal
- Circulatory system
- Mental disorders
- Respiratory system
- Nervous system
- Injury and poisoning
- Signs and symptoms
- Digestive system
- Other

Source: Social Security Statistics 1992

89

(c) Illnesses of men

Lifestyle factors such as smoking, alcohol consumption, poor diet and nutrition, and inadequate physical activity play a major part in the aetiology of cardiovascular and respiratory disease, some cancers and many other conditions which account for much of the burden of morbidity and mortality in men and women alike. The higher prevalence of unhealthy lifestyles, now or in the past, helps to explain why many of these diseases are more common in men (see Figures 4.9-4.13). Initiatives to promote healthier lifestyles should benefit men and women alike, and are discussed elsewhere in this Report. This section therefore highlights diseases and conditions found only in men or which are far commoner among men than women.

Figure 4.9: *Cigarette smoking prevalence by age and sex, Great Britain, 1972-90*

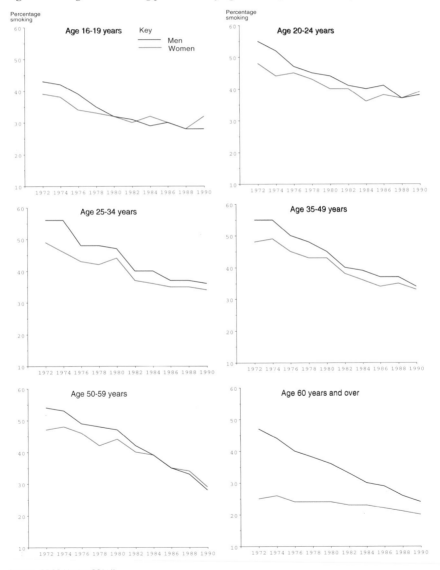

Source: OPCS Monitor SS91/3

90

Figure 4.10: *Alcohol consumption by sex and age, Great Britain, 1990*

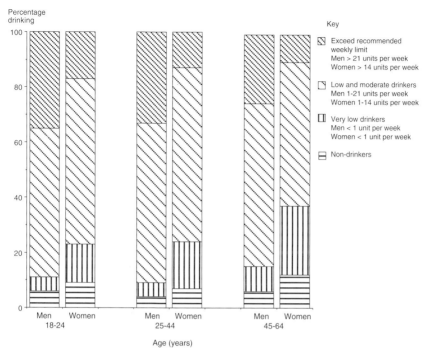

Source: General Household Survey 1990

Figure 4.11: *Percentage of population falling within Committee on Medical Aspects of Food Policy recommendations* for total fat intake, Great Britain, 1986/87*

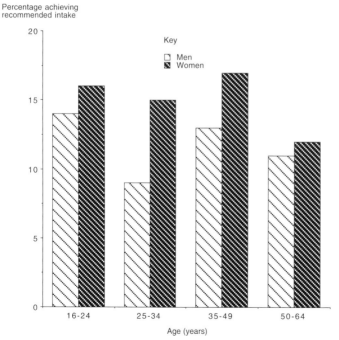

*Individual's total fat intake should not exceed 35% of their food energy.

Source: OPCS, Dietary and Nutritional Survey of British Adults

91

Figure 4.12: *Mean serum total cholesterol* by age and sex, England, 1986/87 and 1991*

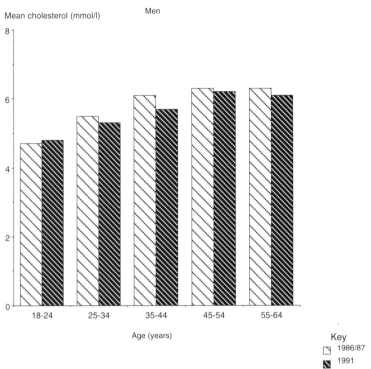

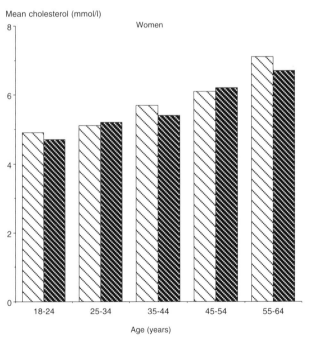

*Excludes persons taking lipid lowering drugs.

Source: OPCS, Dietary and Nutritional Survey of British Adults, 1986/87, and Health Survey for England, 1991

Figure 4.13: *Lack of physical activity* by sex and age, England, 1991*

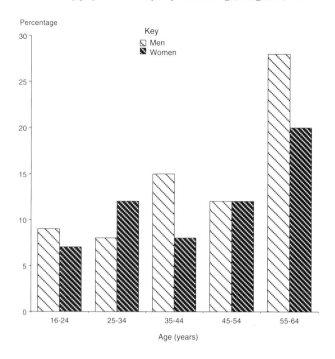

*Percentage of people reporting no physical activity in past 4 weeks, based on number of 20-minute occasions (all activities) of vigorous or moderate or mixed intensity physical activity.

Source: OPCS

(i)   Prostatism and cancer of the prostate

Up to 40% of men aged 65-69 years have clinically detectable benign prostatic hyperplasia. Prostatic hyperplasia becomes progressively more common at later ages (see Figure 4.14). In any individual, however, prostate gland hypertrophy does not necessarily cause a gradual increase in symptoms. Many men present with acute urinary retention: in 1990, 16% of transurethral resections of the prostate (TURPs) and 35% of retropubic prostatectomies (RPPs) were performed as emergency operations[1].

From 1975 to 1990, there was a 62% increase in prostatectomies in National Health Service (NHS) hospitals despite the development of novel interventions such as ultrasound and microwave treatment, as well as new drug regimens. The relations between pathology, clinical findings and symptoms, and how these should influence treatment or might affect outcome, remain unclear. Indeed, operation rates for prostatic disease vary enormously among health Districts - from 2.8 to 29.2 per 10,000 men for TURPs and from 0.08 to 25 per 10,000 for RPPs. Accordingly, the Department of Health (DH) identified benign prostatic hyperplasia as a priority area for research funding in 1993/94.

Figure 4.14: *Recorded incidence of prostatic hyperplasia* at post-mortem*

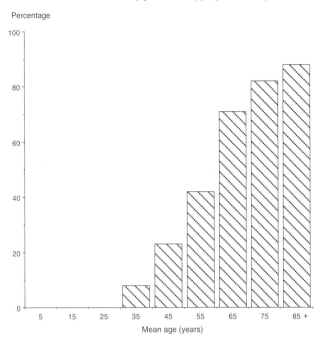

Percentage

Mean age (years)

*As assessed by histological examination of post-mortem specimens; pooled data from several countries, 1943-75.

Source: *J Urol* 1984; **132**: 474-9

Cancer of the prostate is unusual in men under the age of 50 years; the incidence rises thereafter, and it most commonly occurs in men over the age of 70 years. Although the incidence has risen over the past decade (see Figures 4.15 and 4.16), the reasons for this increase are unclear. However, occult carcinoma of the prostate may be found in up to 30% of men over the age of 50 years[2], and these tumours may persist for many years without metastasis[3]. The most appropriate timing of treatment for localised prostate cancer is under debate, and there is still no consensus about the best form of treatment[4]. Radical surgery may lead to impotence or incontinence, radiotherapy to impotence or proctitis, and both forms of treatment may be followed by local or metastatic recurrence.

In about 80% of patients, tumour growth can be suppressed by orchidectomy or anti-androgen therapy, and these treatments can also be used to relieve bone pain from metastatic disease. Total or subcapsular bilateral orchidectomy still has an important place in the management of advanced disease. Oestrogens are also effective but their association with increased cardiovascular mortality has prompted a change to alternatives such as anti-androgens and analogues of luteinising-hormone releasing hormone. Other forms of chemotherapy have only been used in very advanced disease. Radiotherapy can be used for painful metastases and early treatment of the primary tumour. Hormone manipulation may have a greater impact on morbidity rather than mortality: a Medical Research Council (MRC) trial is under way to assess whether it should be introduced early in the disease or only for symptom relief.

Figure 4.15: *Prostate cancer by age: incidence, England and Wales, 1987, and mortality, England, 1992*

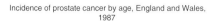

Incidence of prostate cancer by age, England and Wales, 1987

Mortality from prostate cancer by age, England, 1992

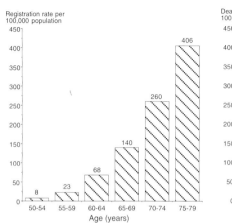

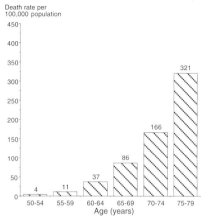

Source: OPCS, MB1 Cancer statistics

Source: OPCS

Figure 4.16: *Prostate cancer by age: time trends in incidence, England and Wales, 1973 and 1987, and mortality, England, 1978 and 1992*

Time trend in incidence of prostate cancer by age, England and Wales, 1973 and 1987

Time trend in mortality from prostate cancer by age, England, 1978 and 1992

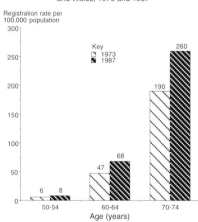

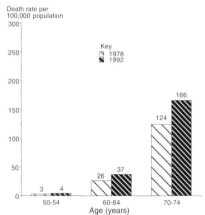

Source: OPCS, MB1 Cancer statistics

Source: OPCS

95

Unfortunately, there is no reliable way to detect early prostatic cancer. Prostatic specific antigen (PSA) has largely replaced acid phosphatase as a marker for prostate cancer[5]. PSA is slightly raised in benign hyperplasia of the prostate but is usually very high in metastatic prostate cancer; however, PSA concentrations may not be raised with poorly differentiated or early tumours. (PSA assays can be used to follow the response to treatment, and increases after surgery indicate the need for a bone scan to look for metastatic disease[6].) Digital examination of the rectum is not sufficiently sensitive to detect early tumours, and the role of ultrasound examination is being assessed. There is also no way to distinguish a tumour likely to remain dormant for years from one that will rapidly progress, and the most appropriate treatment for early prostatic cancer remains unclear. Until these dilemmas are resolved, a comprehensive screening programme (even if a reliable screening test were available) would be ineffective.

(ii) Testicular tumours

Testicular tumours have a peak incidence around the age of 30 years (see Figure 4.17) and are the most common tumours in men aged 20-34 years, but the success of modern treatment regimens means that most patients will be cured. Mortality continues to fall even though the incidence of these tumours has increased over the past decade (see Figure 4.18). However, some testicular tumours grow rapidly and disseminate to the lungs and other organs, and death still occurs.

The two main groups of tumours are seminomas and malignant teratomas. Seminomas can occur at any age, with a median of 35-40 years. At first attendance, 75% have localised tumour. Spread to abdominal lymph nodes can be treated effectively by radiotherapy; more distant metastases are uncommon. Teratomas most commonly occur between 20 and 30 years-of-age; about half are localised at presentation, but teratoma may occasionally present as lung metastases with an undetected small primary tumour. 80% of teratomas secrete chorionic gonadotrophin and alpha fetoprotein: serial measurement of blood concentrations allows the response to treatment, or tumour recurrence, to be monitored[7].

Modern management includes early operation to remove the primary tumour and to diagnose the tumour type, and further investigations to assess the spread of tumour; these factors will determine treatment. Fertility will be affected both by orchidectomy and subsequent chemotherapy, and patients who plan to have a family should also be referred to a sperm bank for evaluation and possible cryopreservation. The prospect of orchidectomy is very unsettling for any young man, and emotional support is often essential at this difficult time.

For patients who present with localised teratoma, cure rates are high and the risk of recurrence is reduced by adjuvant combined chemotherapy. Patients with metastatic disease are usually cured by similar regimens, with cure rates of 69-90%[8] but, if the disease is very bulky or advanced, cure rates are only about 50%[9]. Of men treated successfully for testicular cancer, 2.8% develop a tumour in the other testis[10].

Figure 4.17: *Registrations of malignant neoplasm of testis by age, England and Wales, 1987*

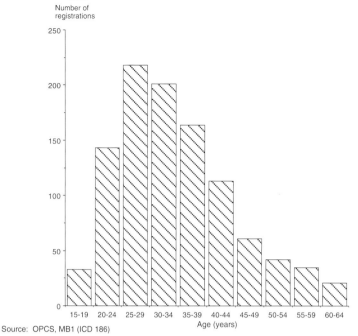

Number of registrations

Age (years)

Source: OPCS, MB1 (ICD 186)

Figure 4.18: *Time trend in registrations for testicular cancer*, England and Wales, 1979-87*

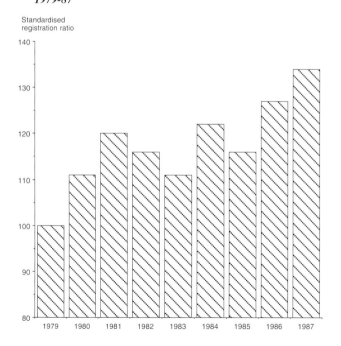

Standardised registration ratio

*Standardised registration ratio allows for changing age structure of population.

Note: 1979 = 100.

Source: OPCS, MB1 (ICD 186)

Men with a history of undescended testicle are at particular risk of testicular cancer. Primary prevention must therefore include examination for (and treatment of) cryptorchidism at pre-school medical examinations: early orchidopexy reduces the risk of testicular atrophy and allows the testis to be more readily examined, but may not prevent the later development of testicular cancer. All men should be encouraged to report any swelling or changes in consistency of a testicle, but men with a history of cryptorchidism need to be particularly aware of the importance of such symptoms.

(iii) X-linked disorders

X-linked diseases tend to be expressed in males, who have one X chromosome, whereas females (who possess two X chromosomes) act as carriers of the disorder. Haemophilia A and B are good examples: in haemophilia A, there is reduced or absent factor VIII, and in haemophilia B, factor IX is similarly affected. Patients with severe haemophilia experience spontaneous joint bleeds; those with mild disease may only have a tendency to prolonged bleeding after trauma or surgery. Some female carriers may have similar symptoms to patients with mild haemophilia. In December 1991, 5,387 patients with haemophilia A and 1,092 with haemophilia B were registered in the UK.

Other X-linked disorders include Duchenne and Becker muscular dystrophy (in which symptoms usually begin at 3-5 years-of-age and death often occurs before adulthood), X-linked retinitis pigmentosa and other eye disorders.

Prevention depends upon identification of female carriers of the particular disorder, so that they may make informed decisions on parenthood, and effective prenatal diagnostic techniques.

(iv) Male infertility

About 15% of all couples seek medical help for infertility[11,12]. In about a quarter of couples investigated, the man is infertile because of deficient sperm production or abnormal sperm structure or motility. There is some evidence[13] that sperm quality in the population as a whole has deteriorated during the past 50 years. There is no effective treatment for most male infertility. The cumulative success rate of donor insemination, if acceptable to a couple, is 75%. Surgical procedures help a small proportion of infertile men and a few can be assisted by electro-ejaculation, or in-vitro fertilisation treatment which may involve micro-manipulation techniques[14]. Cryopreservation of sperm can be offered to men whose reproductive capacity will be compromised or destroyed by surgery, chemotherapy or radiotherapy.

(v) Impotence

Most cases of impotence arise from psychological causes but a physical cause must always be excluded. Androgen deficiency, neurological disorders, diabetes mellitus, radical prostatic surgery and some drug treatments can all lead to impotence. Psychological causes of impotence include excess alcohol intake, depression, anxiety, relationship difficulties, diminished libido and performance anxiety: therapy is usually most effective if directed at the couple, with attention to general relationship issues and risk behaviours.

Treatment of impotence from physical causes is dependent on accurate assessment of what is often a complex clinical problem. Impotence may often be more distressing to the patient than other symptoms of the underlying illness. Treatment options include penile prostheses implanted into the corpora of the penis, and inflatable prostheses that incorporate reservoirs and a pump; intracavernosal injections of vasoactive drugs, such as phentolamine, may be effective in patients with non-vascular causes of impotence.

(vi) HIV/AIDS

Over the past decade, HIV infection has emerged as a substantial contributor to male mortality, particularly among men aged 25-44 years in the four Thames health Regions. To date, most known HIV infections have been acquired as a result of sex between men. In addition, almost all recipients of contaminated blood products have been males with haemophilia, and most injecting drug misusers infected with HIV have been male. Up to the end of 1992, 93% of people with a diagnosis of AIDS and 88% of those infected with HIV have been male. Men are likely to account for most of the HIV epidemic in England for the rest of this century, particularly in view of evidence of continued high-risk behaviour among homosexual men and data from the Government's programme of anonymised HIV surveys (see page 151). These findings, and results from behavioural research[15], strongly indicate a need for continued and targeted educational campaigns to encourage and to sustain behavioural change.

(vii) Other sexually transmitted diseases

For many sexually transmitted diseases, cases in men exceed those in women: for example, males accounted for 68% of cases of infectious syphilis and 61% of cases of gonorrhoea in 1991 (see page 160). The highest incidence occurs among men aged 25-34 years, later than the peak age of incidence in women. Men may be exposed more often to the risk of infection because they tend to have more heterosexual partners than women. However, the figures may be misleading because men are more likely than women to experience symptoms. The proportion of sexually transmitted disease (other than HIV/AIDS) caused by sex between men is also unknown.

(viii) Mental health

There are striking sex differences in the incidence and prevalence of symptoms of mental disorders. Men are only half as likely to have depressive or anxiety symptoms (1.8-7.9% of men compared with 2.7-16.5% of women, dependent on the criteria used), phobic anxiety (4-15% compared with 9-26%), and panic disorder[16]. However the ratio reaches equality in obsessive-compulsive and schizophrenic disorders; for schizophrenia, the peak onset in males occurs much earlier (15-24 years-of-age) than in females (35-39 years-of-age).

The reasons for these disparities are not understood although cultural influences may give rise to differential responses to stress; men may be more likely to resort to substance abuse or antisocial behaviour. GPs seem to be less likely to detect psychological disorder in men than in women, and men are less likely than women to tell a doctor or nurse that they feel anxious or depressed[17]. However, once a psychiatric diagnosis is made, men are more than twice as likely as women to be referred to mental health services[18].

Suicide

Women are twice as likely to become depressed or to commit acts of deliberate self-harm, but 2% of men (compared with 1% of women) die from suicide. This discrepancy is increasing: suicide rates are rising in men but falling in women, particularly among people aged 15-34 years. The methods used also differ: poisoning is commonest in both sexes, but whereas 'liquid or solid substances' predominate in women (43%), a third of men use 'other gases', usually car exhaust fumes; use of violent means is also higher among men[19].

The reasons for these differences are unclear but access to the means of suicide has been established as an influential factor[20]. Social problems, such as unemployment and high divorce rates, have been suggested differentially to affect men[21]. It is interesting to note that countries such as the former West Germany, which have seen striking reductions in the toxicity of exhaust fumes over the past decade, have not seen the rise in young male suicide rates that have occurred elsewhere in the EC.

Homelessness

More than ten times as many men than women are found in surveys of homeless people who use day centres and open access accommodation, and 30-50% are mentally ill. In those who sleep rough, frank mental illness appears to be less common (10%), but substance abuse affects up to 60%.

Learning disabilities

Fragile X syndrome is the second most commonly diagnosed cause of learning difficulties in males. Apart from severe learning disability the syndrome can also be associated with autism. In Klinefelter's syndrome (XXY, with an extra X chromosome), the degree of learning disability varies but is usually mild; often intelligence is within the normal range. Learning disability may also be present in the XYY syndrome (where a man has an extra Y chromosome).

(ix) Accidents

In 1992, there were 4,743 deaths caused by accidental injuries to people in England aged 15-64 years; over three-quarters of these were in men. The rate of accidental death in men exceeds that in women at all ages.

In males, motor vehicle traffic accidents account for 46% of all accidental deaths, whereas in females accidental falls are the commonest cause of death. For traffic accidents among drivers over 40 years-of-age the difference in accident rates between men and women may reflect the greater mileage travelled by men[22]. Nonetheless, whatever the effect of gender in older drivers, young men are much more likely to have accidents than young women when driving[23].

For accidents that are not fatal, estimates based on the Home Accident Surveillance System indicate that, in the UK, males would have had 1,276,000 (49.2%) and females 1,316,000 (50.7%) home accidents in 1990[24]. Although the overall numbers are similar, sex differences between the types of injury have been shown: for example, men more commonly sustain open wounds and fractures than women. Men are also more likely than women to be involved in sporting accidents.

References

1. Donovan J, Frankel S, Nanchahal K, Coast J, Williams M. *Prostatectomy for benign prostatic hyperplasia.* London: Department of Health, 1992 (Epidemiologically based needs assessment; report 8).
2. Kirk D. Prostatic carcinoma. *BMJ* 1985; **290:** 875-7.
3. George NJR. Natural history of localised prostatic cancer managed by conservative therapy alone. *Lancet* 1988; **i:** 494-7.
4. Paulson DF, Lin GH, Hinshaw W, et al for the Uro-Oncology Research Group. Radical surgery versus radiotherapy for adenocarcinoma of the prostate. *J Urol* 1982; **128:** 502-4.
5. Stamey TA, Yang N, Hay AR, John EMcN, Freiha FS, Redwine E. Prostate-specific antigen as a serum marker for adenocarcinoma of the prostate. *N Engl J Med* 1987; **317:** 909-16.
6. Nunan TO, O'Doherty M. Prostate specific antigen and the bone scan. *Nuclear Med Commun* 1992; **13:** 579.
7. Mead GM. Testicular cancer and related neoplasms. *BMJ* 1992; **304:** 1426-9.
8. Ellis M, Sikora K. Mortality in patients with testicular cancer: report of the Anglia and Trent testicular tumour groups. *BMJ* 1986; **292:** 672-4.
9. Bajorin DF. Prognostic classification in metastatic non-seminoma. In: Horwich A, ed. *Testicular cancer: investigation and management.* London: Chapman and Hall, 1991.
10. Von der Maase H, Rørth M, Walbom-Jorgensen S, et al. Carcinoma-in-situ of contralateral testis in patients with testicular germ cell cancer: study of 27 cases in 500 patients. *BMJ* 1986; **293:** 1398-401.
11. Hull MGR, Glazener CMA, Kelly NJ, et al. Population study of causes, treatment and outcome of infertility. *BMJ* 1985; **291:** 1693-7.
12. Templeton A, Fraser C, Thompson B. The epidemiology of infertility in Aberdeen. *BMJ* 1990; **301:** 148-52.
13. Carlsen E, Giwercman A, Keiding N, Skakkebaek NE. Evidence for decreasing quality of semen during past 50 years. *BMJ* 1992; **305:** 609-13.
14. Templeton AA, Drife JO, eds. *Infertility.* London: Springer-Verlag, 1992.
15. Weatherburn P, Hunt AJ, Hickson FCI, Davies PM. *The sexual lifestyles of gay and bisexual men in England and Wales.* London: HMSO, 1992.
16. Paykel EE. Depression in women. *Br J Psychiatry* 1991; **158** (suppl 10): 22-29.
17. Corney R. Sex differences in general practice attendance and help seeking for minor illnesses. *J Psychosomatic Res* 1990: **5:** 525-34.
18. Goldberg D, Huxley P. *Common mental disorders: a biosocial model.* London: Routledge, 1992.
19. Charlton P, Kelly S, Dunnell K, Evans B, Jenkins R, Wallis R. Trends in suicide rates in England and Wales. *Population Trends* (in press).
20. Marzuk PM, Leon AC, Tardiff K, Morgan EB, Stajic M, Mann JJ. The effect of access to lethal methods of injury on suicidal rates. *Arch Gen Psychiatry* 1992; **49:** 451-8.
21. Hawton K. By their own hand. *BMJ* 1992; **304:** 1000.

22. Lockwood C. *If you double your mileage, do you double your accident risk?* In: Department of Transport. *Road Accidents Great Britain 1991.* London: HMSO, 1992.

23. Rolls G, Hall RD, Ingham R, McDonald M. *Accident risk and behavioural patterns of younger drivers.* Basingstoke: AA Foundation for Road Safety Research, 1991.

24. Consumer Safety Unit. *Home and Leisure Accident Research: 1990 Data: Fourteenth Annual Report of the Home Accident Surveillance System.* London: Department of Trade and Industry, 1992.

(d) Men, health and society

(i) Drug and alcohol misuse

Three-quarters of opioid addicts notified to the Home Office, most of whom are heroin misusers, are men[1]. About 75% of drug misusers have a criminal record, usually related to their use of drugs: in 1988, half the drug offenders in the UK were aged between 21 and 29 years, 88% of them being men[1].

While 80% of men and women alike drink alcohol, 7% of men but only 2% of women are heavy drinkers[2]. Again, there is a very strong relation between alcohol and crime, and about one-fifth of convicted prisoners have an alcohol or drug related problem. The reasons for these apparent sex differences in susceptibility to drugs and alcohol are unknown, but may relate partly to social factors. The consequences have obvious social impact: heavy drinking and illegal drug use can lead to serious financial problems, marital and family difficulties, and homelessness.

Drug misuse is not directly associated with violent crime except as a secondary effect of the illegal drug market, but alcohol use and intoxication have strong links with violent behaviour and crime. This relation is complex: many men are never violent when intoxicated with alcohol, and others can be violent without any alcohol use; however, intoxication tends to be associated with disinhibition, risk-taking behaviours, and increased aggression. In the UK, alcohol is implicated as a factor in 50% of homicides, 40% of domestic violence and 20% of child abuse - most of these offences being committed by men[2].

(ii) Violence and mental disorder

In general, women are much less likely to commit a violent offence than men but the gap is decreasing[3]. Most mentally disordered patients who have offended violently are men and many form the greater part of the inpatient population of Regional Secure Units and Special Hospitals. Violence appears to be more commonly associated with some mental disorders than in the general population, but again the picture is complex and requires further clarification[4,5]. However, only a very small minority of mentally disordered men are perpetrators of violent offences and they are responsible for only a tiny fraction of all violence.

(iii) Marital status and mental health

Single, divorced and widowed men have higher rates of mental illness than married men, and married men have lower rates of mental illness than married women. However, single, divorced and widowed men do not have lower rates of mental illness than their female counterparts. The relation of marital status to psychiatric illness is complex, and differs among groups of different educational attainments and social expectations; social isolation, poverty and the presence of children are important factors[6,7,8].

(iv) Health and work

Work patterns have changed dramatically in recent years (see Figure 4.19). Since 1971, there has been a significant fall in employees in manufacturing industries (down by over a third between 1971 and 1990) and an increase in those employed in service industries (up by a third over the same period). Men comprise 13.7 million of the total English workforce of 24 million.

Figure 4.19: *Number of persons in employment by industry, United Kingdom, 1971-90*

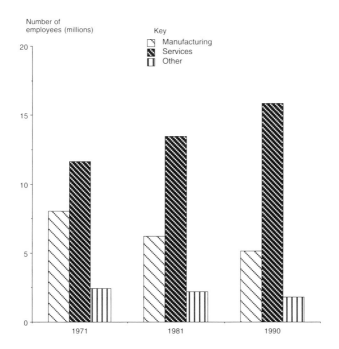

Source: *Social Trends* 1992: **22**

Specific occupations have been identified with special health-related risks. Associations between occupation and carcinogenesis have been appreciated for some time: new cases of bladder cancer in dye workers are now rare, as are those of hepatic angiosarcoma in workers exposed to vinyl chloride. However, mesothelioma in workers exposed to asbestos is still an important occupational neoplasm; other associations include those between employment in foundries, forges and rolling mills, where hot tars and pitches are encountered, and squamous cell carcinomas.

103

Workplace accidents data show that, in 1990/91, 98% of fatal injuries, 75% of major injuries and 78% of 'over 3-day' injuries occurred among men[9]. Distribution of major and 'over 3-day' occupational injuries by age also shows a different pattern for men and women employees; the peak rate in men occurs at 25-34 years-of-age but that in women occurs at 45-54 years-of-age. There are consistently higher injury rates in men in all sectors of employment: the sectors that show the highest injury rates for men are not necessarily the same as those for women, which may reflect sex differences in the types of job undertaken.

Studies of unemployed men indicate that unemployment usually has an adverse effect on health[10,11], even after adjustment for social class and pre-existing morbidity[11,12,13]. Unemployed men are more likely than those still working to die from lung cancer, CHD, pulmonary diseases, accidents and suicide[11,12,13], and have a greater incidence of parasuicide, depression, and anxiety and reduced psychological well-being[14,15,16]. Wives of unemployed men also have increased morbidity and mortality, as do their children[17,18,19], and separation, divorce and family violence are also linked to unemployment[20,21,22].

References

1. National Audit of Drug Misuse Statistics. *Drug misuse in Britain.* London: Institute for Studies of Drug Dependence, 1990.
2. Health Education Authority. *Health Update 3. Alcohol.* London: Health Education Authority, 1992.
3. Home Office. *Statistics of Mentally Disordered Offenders, England and Wales, 1989 and 1990.* London: Home Office, 1991.
4. Taylor PJ, Gunn J. Violence and psychosis I: risk of violence amongst psychiatric men. *BMJ* 1984; **288**: 1945-9.
5. Taylor PJ, Gunn J. Violence and psychosis II: effect of psychiatric diagnosis on conviction and sentencing of offenders. *BMJ* 1984; **289**: 9-12.
6. Meile RL, Johnson DR, St Peter L. Marital role, education, and mental disorder among women: test of an interaction hypothesis. *Health Soc Behaviour* 1976; **17**: 295-301.
7. Pearlin LI, Johnson JS. Marital status, life strains and depression. *Am Sociol Rev* 1977; **42**: 704-15.
8. Cochrane R, Stopes-Roe M. Factors affecting the distribution of psychological symptoms in urban areas of England. *Acta Psychiatr Scand* 1980; **61**: 445-60.
9. Health and Safety Statistics 1990-91. *Employment Gazette* 1992; **100**(9) (Occasional Supplement no. 3).
10. Moser K, Goldblatt PO, Fox J, Jones DR. *Unemployment and mortality.* In: Goldblatt P, ed. *Longitudinal study 1971-1981: mortality and social organisations.* London: HMSO, 1990: 82-96.
11. Moser K, Goldblatt PO, Fox AJ, Jones DR. Unemployment and mortality: comparison of the 1971 and 1981 longitudinal study census samples. *BMJ* 1987; **294:** 86-90.
12. Morris JK. Loss of employment and subsequent mortality. *Proc Soc Social Med* 1992 (suppl A).
13. Cooke DG, Cummins RO, Bartley MJ, Sharpe AG. Health of unemployed middle aged men in Great Britain. *Lancet* 1982; **i:** 1290-4.
14. Smith R. "What's the point, I'm no use to anybody": the psychological consequences of unemployment. *BMJ* 1985; **291:** 1338-41.
15. Platt S, Kreitman N. Long-term trends in parasuicide and unemployment in Edinburgh 1968-87. *Soc Psychol Psychiatr Epidemiol* 1990; **25:** 56-61.
16. Warr PB. *Work, unemployment and mental health.* Oxford: Clarenden Press, 1987.
17. Arber S. Class, paid employment and family roles: making sense of structural disadvantage, gender and health status. *Soc Sci Med* 1991; **32**: 425-36.
18. Brennan ME, Lancashire R. Association of childhood mortality with housing status and unemployment. *J Epidemiol Community Health* 1978; **32:** 28-33.

19. Macfarlane A, Cole T. *From depression to recession - evidence about the effects of unemployment on mothers' and babies' health, 1930s to 1980s.* In: Durward L, ed. *Born unequal: perspectives on pregnancy and childrearing in unemployed families.* London: Maternity Alliance, 1985.

20. Beale N, Nethercott S. Job loss and family mortality: a study of factory closure. *J R Coll Gen Practitioners* 1985; **280**: 510-4.

21. Smith R. "We got on each other's nerves". Unemployment and the family. *BMJ* 1985; **291**: 1707-10.

22. Dew M, Penkower L, Bronet E. Effects of unemployment on mental health in the contemporary family. *Behaviour Modification* 1991; **4:** 501-44.

(e) Improving the health of men

Gender differences in mortality and morbidity undoubtedly exist: but what are they caused by and what can be done about them? There is increasing evidence that many of the patterns observed stem from differences in health-related behaviour, which may be influenced by the knowledge, attitudes and beliefs of men. For example, men seem to be less aware than women of the impact of certain behaviours on their health, such as the types of foods that increase the risk of cardiovascular disease[1], and the increased risk of skin cancer from sun exposure[2]. Similarly, the disproportionate number of motor vehicle accidents among young males appears, at least in part, to be the result of their own perception of their ability to avoid such accidents[3].

Such evidence illustrates the importance of 'behavioural epidemiology' which Raymond has called the basic science that underlies health promotion[4]. Studies of health-related behaviour indicate that considerable gains may be achieved by specific targeting of messages to improve men's general knowledge about health and, more specifically, to improve their awareness of the links between their own behaviour and its health consequences. Unfortunately the same attitudes and behaviours that put men at greater risk also tend to make them less accessible to health promotion messages. Several studies[5,6,7] have shown that men are less ready than women to recognise that they have a health problem, or to seek professional help.

As a result, men seek medical attention less often than women - but tend to die earlier, particularly between the ages of 15 and 64 years[8]. Overall, 70% of people attend their GP at least once each year; of those who do not attend, 66% are men[9]. Habitual non-attenders are unlikely to respond to an invitation for a general health check and also tend not to visit accident and emergency departments or community pharmacies. This pattern of use of health care services causes difficulties for health promotion among men, because there is less scope for opportunistic screening or health counselling. It is also true that many health promotion clinics have been specifically aimed at women; 'well men' clinics are much rarer than 'well women' clinics, and this balance should be reviewed. Men also need to receive health promotion messages in other ways - through the workplace, sporting venues, public houses, male interest magazines and more general media. Despite an apparent indifference, if not resistance, to health promotion messages among men, it must be brought home to them that many of the risk factors to their health - such as smoking, physical inactivity, poor diet, excess alcohol consumption, unsafe sexual practices and risky behaviour likely to lead to accidents - are preventable. Thus the scope for men to improve their health, and to prolong active, healthy life, is considerable.

References

1. Rushworth RL, Plant AJ, Pierce JP, Bauman A, Aldrich R, Cripps AL. The awareness of the risk of elevated cholesterol levels and knowledge about cholesterol-lowering action in Australia. *Med J Aust* 1990; **152**: 72-5.
2. Newman S, Nichols S, Freer C, Izzard L. How much do the public know about moles, skin cancer and malignant melanoma? The results of a postal survey. *Commun Med* 1988; **10:** 351-7.
3. Farrow JA, Brissing PM. Risk for DWI: a new look at gender differences in drinking and driving influences, experiences, and attitudes among new adolescent drivers. *Health Educ Quart* 1990; **17**: 213-21.
4. Raymond JS. Behavioral epidemiology: the science of health promotion. *Health Promotion* 1989; **4:** 281-6.
5. Horwitz A. The pathways into psychiatric treatment: some differences between men and women. *J Health Social Behaviour* 1977; **18**: 169.
6. Nathanson A. Sex, illness and medical care: a review of data theory and method. *Soc Sci Med* 1977; **11**: 13-25.
7. Mechanic D. Effects of psychological distress on perception of physical health and use of medical and psychiatric facilities. *J Hum Stress* 1978; **12**: 26-32**.**
8. Royal College of General Practitioners, Office of Population Censuses and Surveys, Department of Health and Social Security. *1981-1982 Morbidity Statistics from General Practice: Third National Study.* London: HMSO, 1986 (Series MB5; no.1).
9. Thompson KJ, Nichol JP, Fall M, Lowy A, Williams BT. The case against targetting long-term non-attenders in general practice for health checks. *Br J Gen Practice* (in press).

CHAPTER 5

HEALTH CARE

(a) Needs, effectiveness and outcomes

(i) Assessing health care needs

Assessment of local health care needs continues to be a major part of District Health Authority (DHA) activity in preparation for sound contracts with providers of health care. Department of Health (DH) guidance in *Assessing Health Care Needs*[1], the commissioning of a series of epidemiologically based needs reviews, and the setting up of a networking centre through funding of the Birmingham Institute of Public Health were discussed in last year's Report[2]. By December 1992, the series of epidemiological studies of needs assessment comprised the original reports on diabetes mellitus and hip and knee replacement surgery, and further reports on stroke[3], renal disease[4], dementia[5], mental illness[6], alcohol misuse[7], prostatectomy for benign prostatic hyperplasia[8], varicose vein treatments[9], coronary heart disease (CHD)[10], cancer of the lung[11], learning disabilities[12], hernia repair[13], and cataract surgery[14]. More topics will be covered during 1993.

The assessment of health care needs is now also a function of local authority social services departments and of Family Health Services Authorities (FHSAs) in their assessments of social and primary care requirements, respectively. DH, in conjunction with Price Waterhouse, has assembled guidance for local authorities which will be published in 1993. An important message will be that such assessments should consider not only the incidence and prevalence of disease but also the ability of health or social services to cope with disease; effectiveness of care is a vital part of needs assessment (see page 110).

A major contribution to the quantification of local disease burdens has been made by development of the *Public Health Common Data Set*, available as 14 regional volumes, and as a selected and illustrated national volume[15]. Data on demography, fertility, and mortality, and available information on morbidity and risk factors are set out for Regional Health Authorities (RHAs) and DHAs. In 1992, the Data Set[16] was extended to include baseline indices for specific targets in the strategy for health[17], by DHA, as well as an analysis of trends in mortality.

(ii) Basic sources of information

During 1992, considerable progress was made in the development of novel or improved sources of information and of the means for processing such information.

The health survey programme

The 1991 Health Survey for England yielded interviews (and in most cases measurements) from approximately 3,250 adults, with adequate blood samples obtained from a subgroup of about 2,300; a full report on the 1991 survey will be published in 1993. Fieldwork for the 1992 survey has been completed and a report is expected early in 1994. The 1993 survey will be larger, with a sample size of approximately 17,000 adults, but otherwise this and the 1992 survey will follow a similar pattern to that in 1991, apart from minor modifications such as the addition of blood analysis for fibrinogen, gamma glutamyltransferase, glycosylated haemoglobin, and cotinine. From 1995 onwards, the survey will probably be extended to take into account other priority areas that arise from the strategy for health[17]. But local as well as national assessments of health and health needs are essential: it is hoped to set up a National Health Service (NHS) Survey Advice Centre to provide advice, support and training for local surveys related to health, and to ensure the comparability of methods used in such surveys.

The programme of Dietary and Nutritional Surveys, sponsored jointly with the Ministry of Agriculture, Fisheries and Food (MAFF), also continued. Fieldwork for the first survey, on pre-school children, started in September 1992, and should be completed in August 1993; a report is expected in mid-1994. Plans for a survey of the diet of elderly people are being prepared.

The pilot study for the National Psychiatric Morbidity Survey was successfully completed; the methods used were found to be feasible and acceptable and the main survey will take place in the Summer of 1993, with results available approximately one year later.

Morbidity Statistics from General Practice

The 4th national study of Morbidity Statistics from General Practice collected data from 60 general practices and 500,000 patients for the year to the end of August 1992. Morbidity data were collected for each consultation during the year; socio-economic data were collected separately, with a response rate of over 80% of all registered patients. Preliminary results will be available in the Autumn of 1993 and a full report will be published during 1994.

Public Health Information Strategy

Knowledge may be priceless, but its acquisition can be expensive. DH must ensure that it collects the information required to support its objectives in the most cost-effective way, and has set up a Public Health Information Strategy programme to review the scope of its public health activities; the types of information required to support these activities; and existing information sources and their ability to support these activities. The main inadequacies in data collection have now been identified and a series of projects, guided by the priorities of the strategy for health[17], have been implemented.

Information management and technology

An information management and technology strategy for the NHS in England was launched by the NHS Management Executive in December 1992[18]. It provides for a common infrastructure for information management and technology to support the capture and secure sharing of person-based information. This programme requires the re-issuing of computer-compatible NHS numbers, the definition and coding of common clinical terms, the development of an NHS-wide networking capability and the provision of strict protocols to ensure confidentiality and security. Other initiatives include the setting up of a working group on the sharing of general practitioners' (GPs') morbidity data, the development of prototype clinical workstations and a health information workstation for public health doctors, and an agreement to set up a 'scoping' study into the electronic patient record. The objective of the 'scoping' study, which is headed by a steering group of clinicians, is to determine priorities for the component parts of the electronic patient record.

Clinical terms project

A project to develop a thesaurus of coded, nationally agreed clinical terms and groupings, expanding on the Read Codes used in primary care[19], was set up by the NHS Management Executive and the medical and other health care professions in April 1992. Forty working groups will consider ways to ensure that clinical information - including signs, symptoms, diagnoses and prescribed medications - can be translated and understood on computers across the NHS. The work of the individual working groups will be co-ordinated and in due course combined to produce a comprehensive thesaurus by mid-1994.

(iii) National confidential enquiries

Confidential enquiry is a form of clinical audit that includes scrutiny of other factors which might influence the quality and outcome of care. Its purpose is to improve understanding of the elements that contribute to a particular health outcome, and to identify how the risks of an unfavourable outcome could be reduced, if not avoided. The avenues of investigation include not only risk factors, but also the appropriateness, accessibility and quality of care and service provision.

Enquiries are conducted by independent assessors appointed for their specialist knowledge and experience in a field relevant to the particular enquiry. Inevitably, they require access to confidential personal health information and to information which might reflect the judgments and actions of professionals and managers. A successful enquiry requires secure arrangements to ensure that confidentiality is maintained and that there can be no feedback on individual cases to patients or their relatives.

There are now five national confidential enquiries. The Confidential Enquiry into Maternal Deaths, established in 1952, and the Confidential Enquiry into

Perioperative Deaths, established in 1987, have both made major contributions towards improvements in training, clinical practice and the quality of service provision in their respective fields. During 1992, three further enquiries were established - Stillbirths and Deaths in Infancy (see page 128), Counselling for Genetic Disorders, and Homicides and Suicides by Mentally Ill People. It is expected that they will also make significant contributions towards improved outcomes.

(iv) Quality of service and effectiveness of care

The increase in clinical audit activity continued during 1992: DH allocated £42 million to hospital and community health services audit, over £11 million to audit in primary care and over £7 million to nursing and therapy professional audit. One of the main aims of these programmes is to ensure a permanent place for audit within the health care system.

A key component in demonstrating quality of clinical care is identifying its benefit in terms of improved health, patient satisfaction and improved quality of life - ie clinical outcome. Clinical outcome usually reflects the collective efforts of a number of professionals, and while early audit programmes were set up by different professional groups, there is now a need to move to a more integrated approach[20]. During 1992, the Chief Medical and Nursing Officers took an important step by jointly establishing the Clinical Outcomes Group (COG) to give strategic direction to the move from uniprofessional to multiprofessional clinical audit. The membership of COG reflects a diverse range of disciplines and interests, and the public is also represented by two lay members. COG is actively examining the implications of multiprofessional audit, management aspects, the development of a national clinical quality centre, and the development of audit in primary care and between different sectors of care (interface audit).

Bulletins on the effectiveness of treatments for subfertility[21] and for persistent glue ear in children[22] were published, and similar assessments for the management of depression in primary care and cholesterol screening are in preparation. Eight other effectiveness bulletins were commissioned by DH from a consortium of the Nuffield Institute for Health at Leeds University, the Centre for Health Economics at York University, and the Royal College of Physicians' Research Unit. Topics for review are chosen on the basis of high resource implications, or uncertainty about the efficacy of interventions or their likely impact on health.

(v) Outcomes of care

The assessment of health outcomes of care is now established as a priority within the NHS. The 1991 Report[23] outlined definitions and some central initiatives to take this concept forward, particularly the establishment of the Central Health Outcomes Unit and the United Kingdom (UK) Clearing House on Outcomes, the development of outcome indicators and the setting up of an outcomes research and development programme. Progress continued during 1992.

UK Clearing House on Outcomes

A call for information on outcomes projects led to some 500 responses, which have now been entered onto a structured database alongside entries from published research. A newsletter and a bulletin listing new entries, and criteria for critical appraisal of published work on outcomes, are under preparation.

Population health outcome indicators

The Faculty of Public Health Medicine was commissioned by DH to undertake a feasibility study of potential population health outcome indicators. In the first phase of this study, the Faculty reviewed 21 topics including the justifications for avoidable death indicators. The reviews covered aspects such as effectiveness of interventions; health outcome objectives; definitions of indicators, and their numerators and denominators; sources of data and their reliability; and interpretation of indicators and the extent to which they reflected health care in the context of wider influences. DH commissioned the University of Surrey to undertake a further analysis of 35 indicators recommended by the Faculty, and hopes to publish these in a consultation document, alongside the Faculty's report, during 1993.

Outcomes research and development programme

Health outcome of health care is the health consequence of health services intervention or its lack[23]; DH has identified eight steps for its assessment. Expectation of outcome must be defined by:

- assessment of baseline health status, disease severity and health determinants;

- awareness of the effectiveness and cost-effectiveness of interventions;

- establishment of the health outcome objective of intervention;

- quantification of the health target (over a specified period of time) if appropriate; *and*

- setting standards of health service delivery required to achieve the optimum health outcome of intervention.

These must be followed by steps to audit the success of intervention by:

- audit of health service delivery to the standards specified;

- audit of end-point health status; *and*

- confirmation that end-point health status can be truly attributed to health service intervention (ie, health outcome of health care).

During 1992, the Central Health Outcomes Unit prepared the framework for a structured research and development programme by analysis of the NHS's current ability to perform each of these tasks, by identification of gaps and, where necessary, by support of studies and projects to establish appropriate methods and systems over the next few years.

References

1. Department of Health: NHS Management Executive. *Assessing health care needs.* London: Department of Health, 1991.
2. Department of Health. *On the State of the Public Health: the annual report of the Chief Medical Officer of the Department of Health for the year 1991.* London: HMSO, 1992; 78.
3. Wade DT. *Stroke.* London: Department of Health, 1992 (Epidemiologically based needs assessment; report 3).
4. Beech R, Gulliford M, Mays N, Melia J. *Renal disease.* London: Department of Health, 1992 (Epidemiologically based needs assessment; report 4).
5. Melzer D, Hopkins S, Pencheon D, Brayne C, Williams R. *Dementia.* London: Department of Health, 1992 (Epidemiologically based needs assessment; report 5).
6. Wing JK. *Mental illness.* London: Department of Health, 1992 (Epidemiologically based needs assessment; report 6).
7. Edwards G, Unnithan S. *Alcohol misuse.* London: Department of Health, 1992 (Epidemiologically based needs assessment; report 7).
8. Donovan J, Frankel S, Nanchahal K, Coast J, Williams M. *Prostatectomy for benign prostatic hyperplasia.* London: Department of Health, 1992 (Epidemiologically based needs assessment; report 8).
9. Robbins M, Frankel S, Nanchahal K, Coast J, Williams M. *Varicose vein treatments.* London: Department of Health 1992 (Epidemiologically based needs assessment; report 9).
10. Langham S, Normand C, Piercy J, Rose G. *Coronary heart disease.* London: Department of Health, 1992 (Epidemiologically based needs assessment; report 10).
11. Sanderson H, Mountney L, Harris J. *Cancer of the lung.* London: Department of Health, 1992 (Epidemiologically based needs assessment; report 11).
12. Felce D, Taylor D, Wright K. *People with learning disabilities.* London: Department of Health, 1992 (Epidemiologically based needs assessment; report 12).
13. Williams M, Frankel S, Nanchahal K, Coast J, Donovan J. *Hernia repair.* London: Department of Health, 1992 (Epidemiologically based needs assessment; report 13).
14. Frankel S, Coast J, Nanchahal K, Williams M, Donovan J. *Cataract surgery.* London: Department of Health, 1992 (Epidemiologically based needs assessment; report 14).
15. Institute of Public Health, Department of Health. *Public Health Common Data Set (based on data for years up to 1991): 1992.* Guildford (University of Surrey, Guildford GU2 5XH): Institute of Public Health, 1992.
16. Institute of Public Health, Department of Health. *Public Health Common Data Set: The Health of the Nation baseline data: data definitions and user guide for computer files: 1992.* Guildford (University of Surrey, Guildford GU2 5XH): Institute of Public Health, 1992.
17. Department of Health. *The Health of the Nation: a strategy for health in England.* London: HMSO, 1992 (Cm. 1986).
18. Department of Health. *Tom Sackville launches strategy to improve use of computers in NHS.* London: Department of Health, 1992 (Press Release: H92/447).
19. Chisholm J. The Read clinical classification. *BMJ* 1990; **300:** 1092.
20. Standing Medical Advisory Committee. *The quality of medical care: report of the Standing Medical Advisory Committee.* London: HMSO, 1990.
21. Freemantle N, Ibbotson S, Long A, et al. Management of subfertility. *Effective Health Care* 1992; **3:** 1-24.
22. Freemantle N, Long A, Mason J, et al. The treatment of persistent glue ear in children. *Effective Health Care* 1992; **4:** 1-16.
23. Department of Health. *On the State of the Public Health: the annual report of the Chief Medical Officer of the Department of Health for the year 1991.* London. HMSO, 1992; 81.

(b) Primary health care

(i) *Effects of the new contract*

1992 was a year of further consolidation by primary health care teams after introduction of the new GP contract in 1990[1]. It is sometimes easy to overlook the fact that about 90% of all contacts between patients and health services take place in the primary care setting: the implications for service delivery and patients' satisfaction with those services are obvious, and the opportunities for active intervention in primary care are increasingly recognised. A continued expansion of effective co-operation across the wider primary health care team, which includes pharmacists, optometrists, dentists and other community health professionals, is essential for delivery of the best possible primary health care. Further progress was made during the year - helped by the concept of 'healthy alliances' as promulgated by the strategy for health White Paper[2] and *Caring for People*[3].

Development of primary health care teams continued, with 9,121 nurses employed in general practice in October 1992, nearly 4% more than in October 1991. There were also 169 counsellors helping patients to cope with stress and some mental disorders - the first time figures have been collected for this group - and more than 80,000 ancillary staff. The primary health care nursing task force considers that the overall standard of such nursing care is improving[4]. Indeed, improvements in delivery of primary health care throughout general practice continued within the framework set by the 1990 contract. Following on from last year, the percentage of GPs who achieved the higher targets for childhood immunisation and cervical screening continued to increase. In October, vaccination against *Haemophilus influenzae* type b (Hib) meningitis was introduced, and will be included in immunisation targets after an initial catch-up period.

Health promotion is a vital part of health care and lies at the core of the strategy for health[2]. However, the continued rapid growth in the numbers of GP health promotion clinics has been checked until systems are in place to analyse the benefits of such clinics systematically. The realisation that good practice is driven by good information has led to widespread computerisation within general practice: in 1992, almost £27 million were invested in computers. Good data systems are essential to successful audit, good prescribing, effective health promotion for the registered population and screening, as well as for standard record-keeping to ensure the optimum organisation and delivery of routine demand-led care.

The number of minor surgical procedures remunerated through the contract grew by 30% between 1991 and 1992: over 70% of family doctors now offer these convenient local services to patients. DH set up a working group with representatives from various professional bodies, including the Royal College of General Practitioners (RCGP), the Royal College of Surgeons of England and the British Medical Association (BMA), to develop training and education in minor surgery.

(ii) The strategy for health

In early 1992, DH and the BMA began a series of negotiations that were intended to put health promotion in primary health care on a more scientific footing. Although there was much worthwhile activity in this field, the arrangements were uneven and their benefits hard to quantify. It was agreed that health promotion work would be most effective if directed in support of the objectives of the strategy for health[2]. The meetings laid an agreed foundation for change, to begin in 1993, based on preventive activity for CHD and stroke. The primary health care setting also provides considerable opportunities for prevention of mental illness, and DH is funding a number of initiatives to take forward health promotion in the mental illness key area of the strategy for health[2], including funding of a model to develop optimum primary care for mental illness and to audit that process[5].

Payments for health promotion under the existing arrangements included activity more related to chronic disease management of conditions such as diabetes mellitus and asthma. Care for these conditions is too important to be left to chance and the new arrangements will distinguish such activities from health promotion, whilst retaining much of the good practice that has grown up. Treatment of chronic diseases based on agreed shared-care guidelines should continue and develop.

About 98% of the population are registered with a GP and general practice therefore provides a solid foundation for the delivery of many areas of health care. A working group with representatives from the BMA, RCGP and DH has developed guidelines for programmes to empower patients to make healthier lifestyle choices, and a document entitled *Better Living, Better Life* will be distributed to all general practices early in 1993. Through the King's Fund, DH has sponsored a community oriented primary care project to develop a programme to teach new skills in population medicine to primary health care teams; a report is expected in 1993.

(iii) Prescribing

Since 1981/82, the cost of drugs prescribed by GPs has risen by 166% in cash terms and by almost 50% allowing for inflation. The drugs bill has grown even faster than overall NHS expenditure; the net ingredient cost increased by more than 12% in 1991/92, and the total cost exceeded £2,300 million. The annual number of prescription items per head for patients over retirement age increased from 13 in 1980 to 18 in 1990, and this trend has continued.

There are genuine pressures and good reasons for increased prescribing, including health promotion initiatives to support the strategy for health[2] and the introduction of novel drug therapies. But there is a limit to what the NHS can afford. In 1992, an NHS multidisciplinary Prescribing Task Force began to identify the factors underlying these increases in prescribing, with the aim of helping GPs to adopt more rational prescribing habits. Although interactions in prescribing are complex, the Task Force considers that good prescribing can be economical, and that high cost is no guarantee of quality. Support for such beliefs has been provided by GP fundholders, who have achieved 10% lower prescribing costs, and lower growth in these costs. Some of this success is attributable to more widespread prescribing by generic names.

DH initiatives to encourage high-quality but cost-effective prescribing continue. The indicative prescribing scheme was backed up in 1992 with a new information service - PACTLINE - which analyses prescribing information to enable FHSA and RHA advisers to provide better information for local prescribers. The software produces graphic images of prescribing trends within and between practices, FHSAs and Regions. FHSAs have employed pharmaceutical advisers in greater numbers - a move widely welcomed by practices, and one which has enabled medical advisers to take on a broader range of work in support of service development.

DH has also provided funds for the RCGP to take forward continuing education about mental illness in primary care, which will include analysis of appropriate prescribing. Benzodiazepines, for example, are still widely prescribed for depression and anxiety even though they are not curative and have potential for addiction; given the availability of better forms of treatment, the rate of benzodiazepine prescription remains a cause for concern.

(iv) Clinical audit

The setting up of Medical Audit Advisory Groups in 1991 was followed up by extensive clinical audit activity during 1992. Up to 90% of practices are now involved in clinical audit - a process stimulated by the provision of appropriate training, audit support staff, the construction of databases, and local meetings. Benefits of audit are being seen in various aspects of primary care, including the setting of clinical standards, review of the quality of medical records, and improved team communication and identification of educational needs.

In addition to local initiatives, nearly 200 centrally funded primary care clinical audit projects covered key areas in the strategy for health[2]; other NHS priorities such as prescribing, care in the community, and the integration of primary and secondary care; the management of chronic diseases such as asthma and diabetes mellitus; patient satisfaction; and child health surveillance.

(v) GP fundholding

A second wave of 1,443 GPs in 253 practices became fundholders in April 1992, which meant that 14% of the population were then registered with fundholding practices. During the year many more practices began the preparations necessary to enter the scheme - an encouraging sign of commitment to the success of this initiative. Fundholders continue to be innovative. For example, they have arranged better local access for their patients to services such as counselling, physiotherapy, and consultant outpatient clinics within their practices.

The next big challenge is to develop a shared agenda for patient care with other purchasers, and to incorporate DHAs' public health requirements. Alongside this is the need to find ways to help smaller practices join the scheme. Often this goal can best be achieved by several practices teaming up to share the benefits of fundholding. Learning to work together is not easy for separate practices, cutting across traditions of independence. Five FHSAs and one DHA have begun a project, acting as a management agency, to encourage and to develop such co-operation. A surprising lesson has been that practices do not need to be geographically close together for fundholding to succeed: it seems that effective teamwork is not a function of size or location, but of motivation and a common desire to improve patients' health care.

(vi) Professional development

The vocational training scheme provides the bedrock for quality in general practice. It is the duty of all professional people to keep up to date with new developments. The postgraduate education allowance (PGEA) system supports this and it is encouraging to find that 93.5% of family doctors attended at least 10 sessions of postgraduate education during 1992. The PGEA system seems to provide a good general framework for personal development, but there may be a need to give more structured help to some practitioners.

GPs, as employers, are responsible for ensuring continued education for practice staff, and FHSAs should support GPs in further development of practice nurse training programmes. Time management is increasingly important and practice workloads should be analysed critically to plan delivery of care, optimum use of all staff and time for professional development.

(vii) The way ahead

Recent years have seen striking advances in the level of sophistication of the health care that can now be delivered effectively in the community. The movement of managed care from the hospital sector has been made possible by the interest and dedication of primary health care teams. This widening range of primary care must be accompanied by quality checks and safeguards in the form of good and agreed guidelines for care and meticulous clinical audit.

A comprehensive primary care service needs to reach the whole population. Not all doctors are skilled or comfortable in dealing with people with HIV infection or who misuse drugs, but the availability of satisfactory services must be ensured for everyone - including the 2% who are not registered with any general practice.

The strategy for health[2] reinforces the emphasis on prevention in primary care. Traditional medical education does not provide for the acquisition of skills in population medicine that are needed to deliver proactive care to the whole community. A greater appreciation of epidemiology and health economics might contribute to the achievement of the greatest possible health gain with resources - of people, premises, technology and money - which must inevitably have limits.

References

1. Department of Health. *General Practice: the new contract.* London: Department of Health, 1989 (Executive Letter: EL(89)S/8).
2. Department of Health. *The Health of the Nation: a strategy for health in England.* London: HMSO, 1992 (Cm. 1986).
3. Department of Health. *Caring for People: community care the next decade and beyond.* London: HMSO, 1989 (Cm. 849).
4. Department of Health. *New World, New Opportunities. Report of joint NHS/NHSME Task Force Group on nursing in primary health care.* London: HMSO, 1992.
5. Jenkins R. Developments in the primary care of mental illness - a look forward. *Int Rev Psychiatry* 1992; **4:** 237-42.

(c) Hospital services

(i) *Supra-Regional and Regional Services*

The provision of specialised services continued to be a major topic of debate within the NHS in 1992, and during the year there was a striking increase in the number of enquiries from provider units about the mechanism for applying for the status of a Supra-Regional Service.

Newly designated Supra-Regional Services comprised a new service for proton treatment of large uveal melanomas and two further units for organ transplantation - a heart unit at Queen Elizabeth Hospital, Birmingham and a liver unit at Freeman Hospital, Newcastle. From the end of March 1992, spinal injuries services were withdrawn from the Supra-Regional arrangements.

During 1992 some RHAs introduced arrangements to devolve many of the clinical services previously managed on a Regional basis to local purchasers at District level. Nevertheless, as mentioned in last year's Report[1], many DHAs will have only a small number of patients with uncommon clinical conditions, and to determine a local need for appropriate services is a demanding task. In view of the likely problems of urgent tertiary referrals, the NHS Management Executive issued guidance on new arrangements to address the potential problem of 'cost shifting' between provider units[2].

(ii) *Access and availability*

1992 was the first full year of work for the Clinical Standards Advisory Group, set up in 1991 as part of the NHS reforms to act as an independent source of expert advice to Health Ministers and the NHS on standards of clinical care, and access to and availability of services. The Group's first report, assessing access to and the availability of selected specialist services in the first 18 months after the reforms, will be published in the summer of 1993. It is likely to conclude that this interval was insufficient for the internal market to have significantly affected services for neonatal intensive care, cystic fibrosis, childhood leukaemia and coronary artery bypass grafting, but will point to several potential dangers and make suggestions about how these might be tackled. The Group has a number of other reports in preparation, including studies of emergency and urgent admissions to hospital, pressure sores, and services for people with diabetes mellitus.

(iii) *Cancer*

After CHD, cancers are the most common cause of death in England, accounting for about 25% of deaths in 1992. The Government's long-term objective to reduce the morbidity and mortality caused by all cancers is reflected in the strategy for health White Paper[3], in which specific targets are set for four cancers (lung, breast, cervix and skin; see page 68).

Oncology specialists are usually based in large centres with facilities for radiotherapy, but visit District General Hospitals (DGHs) to hold combined clinics with local specialists to advise on treatment. Nevertheless, a suspected diagnosis of cancer, which may arise from abnormalities detected in the national screening programmes for breast and cervical cancer, usually leads to referral to a specialist assessment centre to establish a diagnosis. In 1992, DH allocated £13.5 million for the purchase of 26 mammography machines, 10 computed tomography (CT) scanners and 6 magnetic resonance imaging (MRI) scanners.

Curative or palliative treatment for any form of cancer may be by surgery, radiotherapy or chemotherapy, singly or in combination. Although chemotherapy may be given in a DGH, radiotherapy is normally confined to larger centres. Surgery for many tumours is often carried out in a DGH, but surgery for some tumours (eg lung cancer) requires referral to Regional centres. Laser palliative treatment for bronchial, oesophageal and rectal tumours is also available in a few hospitals. There are now six Supra-Regional centres for treatment of rare tumours: two each for primary bone tumours and choriocarcinoma, and one each for retinoblastoma and large uveal melanomas (see page 117). In advanced disease, palliative care may be managed in the primary sector.

In 1992, DH allocated £6.5 million for the purchase of linear accelerators and £0.5 million to support a Medical Research Council (MRC) study of continuous hyperfractionated accelerated radiotherapy for head and neck or bronchial tumours; it also commissioned work from two centres to provide manuals on total quality management appraisal in radiotherapy. The high incidence of, and the variety of treatments for, cancer require good record management, and a new minimum data set for registration of cancer will be used from mid-1993.

(iv) Palliative care

In November, DH and the Cancer Relief Macmillan Fund sponsored the European Conference on Palliative Care. The Standing Medical and the Standing Nursing and Midwifery Advisory Committees presented their report *The Principles and Provision of Palliative Care*[4], which recommends that palliative care should be available for all patients and carers who need it, whatever the cause of their terminal illness, and advocates education of all staff required to provide it. 1992 also saw the establishment of the National Council for Hospice and Specialist Palliative Care Services, which co-ordinates the policies of charitable organisations and NHS units, represents their views to Government, and issues guidance about purchaser/provider contracts and community care.

References

1. Department of Health. *On the State of the Public Health: the annual report of the Chief Medical Officer of the Department of Health for the year 1991.* London: HMSO, 1992; 111.
2. NHS Management Executive. *Tertiary referrals.* London: Department of Health, 1992 (Executive Letter: EL (92)97).
3. Department of Health. *The Health of the Nation: a strategy for health in England.* London: HMSO, 1992 (Cm. 1986).
4. Standing Medical Advisory Committee/Standing Nursing and Midwifery Standing Committee. *The principles and provision of palliative care.* London: HMSO, 1992.

(d) Diabetes mellitus

The St Vincent Declaration on diabetes care and research in Europe has set goals and 5-year targets to improve the quality of life and life expectancy of people with diabetes mellitus, and to reduce the number of serious complications caused by the disease[1]. The principles of the Declaration and its recommendations were accepted by Health Ministers and are referred to in the strategy for health[2].

In July 1992, Ministers announced the setting up of a joint DH/British Diabetic Association Task Force to "advise on which aspects of the St Vincent recommendations need to be addressed in England and their relative priority, and to provide detailed advice on the action needed to implement those priority areas agreed with the Department of Health". Chaired by Professor David Shaw, this Task Force is a multidisciplinary group which includes a diabetologist, a general practitioner, a specialist diabetes nurse, a patient who has diabetes, a service purchaser, a service provider, and an epidemiologist. A working party has been set up to look at the data available and at what other information may be needed to monitor improvements in diabetes care. The Task Force will report in 1993 on priorities for further work.

References

1. Diabetes Mellitus in Europe: a problem at all ages in all countries: a model for prevention and self care: a meeting organised by WHO and IDF Europe: proceedings. *Giornale Italiano di Diabetologia* 1990; 10 (suppl).
2. Department of Health. *The Health of the Nation: a strategy for health in England.* London: HMSO, 1992 (Cm. 1986).

(e) Osteopathy

The report of the King's Fund Working Party on Osteopathy, chaired by Lord Justice Bingham, was published in December 1991[1]. The report set out recommendations for the statutory regulation of osteopaths and contained a draft Bill which Lord Walton, a member of the Working Party, introduced into the House of Lords as a Private Peer's Bill on 17 December 1991. The Bill received a Second Reading and successfully completed its Committee stage during 1992, but fell when Parliament was prorogued for the general election.

In June 1992, Mr Malcolm Moss MP introduced a Private Member's Bill into the House of Commons which seeks to establish a General Osteopathic Council to develop, promote and regulate the profession of osteopathy throughout the UK and to set educational standards and standards of professional conduct. The Bill is likely to receive its Second Reading early in 1993.

The King's Fund Working Party on Chiropractic is expected to report in the first half of 1993.

Reference

1. King Edward's Hospital Fund for London. *Report of working party on osteopathy.* London : King Edward's Hospital Fund for London, 1991. Chair: Lord Justice Bingham.

(f) Mental health

(i) *Care Programmes, Specific Grant, and central London homeless mentally ill initiative*

Evaluation of the implementation of the Care Programme Approach[1] was commissioned and a report will be circulated in 1993. The funding of the mental illness Specific Grant was increased by 9% to £34.4 million, supporting expenditure of £49.1 million.

The third phase of the Homeless Mentally Ill Initiative for homeless people sleeping rough in central London was announced in January 1992. By the end of 1992, it included four specialist hostels and five multidisciplinary community psychiatric teams who actively seek out homeless people with mental illness and encourage them into specialist accommodation or more standard psychiatric services.

(ii) *Development of brief rating scales for mental health*

The first target in the mental illness key area of the strategy for health[2] is "to improve significantly the health and social functioning of mentally ill people". To monitor progress towards this target, it is necessary to be able to measure health and social functioning objectively and directly. Techniques to do so are already used in psychiatric research, but are too lengthy for routine use in clinical settings. The Royal College of Psychiatrists was therefore commissioned to lead the multidisciplinary development of brief rating scales that can be used in routine clinical work to measure health, social functioning and quality of life, and to conduct pilot studies of their use.

(iii) *Psychiatric morbidity survey*

To improve the understanding of mental health needs in the general population, DH commissioned a national psychiatric survey from the Office of Population Censuses and Surveys (OPCS). This study will provide baseline data on the prevalence of mental illness in the population, and associated disabilities, risk factors and use of services. A pilot study in the summer of 1992 showed that the methods used were feasible and acceptable. The full survey, to start in 1993, will comprise four key elements:

- a survey of private households;

- a survey of residents in communal establishments that cater specifically for people with mental illness;

- a survey of people with known severe mental illness to improve knowledge about their use of services; *and*

- a survey of people in temporary accommodation or who sleep in the open (to ensure that prevalence estimates do not exclude homeless people).

(iv) Mental health and primary care

One in three people who consult their GP have a demonstrable psychosocial component to the consultation, but such a problem is identified in only one in six attenders[3]. Recognised psychiatric morbidity accounts for 30,000-40,000 such contacts annually per 500,000 people. Thus, a further 30,000-40,000 consultations represent 'hidden' psychiatric morbidity. Furthermore, patients with recognised psychiatric morbidity who consult their GPs outnumber outpatient attenders at consultant clinics by a factor of 10, and psychiatric admissions by a factor of 100[4].

Only 35-50% of patients with schizophrenia are in contact with mental health services, only a small proportion of problem drinkers in the community are known to specialised agencies, and elderly people with dementia are likely to present first to their GP[2]. Nevertheless, depression and anxiety are the commonest mental illnesses in primary care. 5% of GP attenders have major depression, 5% have mild depression and a further 10% have clear depressive symptoms[5]. Groups at increased risk of depression include the elderly, mothers with small children, people with chronic physical illness, the disabled, the bereaved, the socially isolated and those who are blind or deaf. It must be emphasised that 90% of people who commit suicide have some form of mental disorder, especially depression: 66% will have seen their GP in the previous month (40% in the past week) and a third will have expressed clear suicidal intent[3]. Achievement of mental health targets in the strategy for health[2] (see page 70) will therefore require a considerable contribution from primary care.

In 1992, DH was involved in a number of initiatives to improve the primary care of mental illness. Conferences were organised on counselling[6] and primary care of schizophrenia[7]. Projects were funded from the National Development Fund, including evaluation of GP facilitators and a 'model' general practice to develop the best possible primary care for mental illness. A senior RCGP Fellowship has also been established to take a national lead on mental health education in general practice[4].

(v) Occupational mental health

'You don't have to be mad to work here, but it helps'. Alas, mental health in the workplace is an important issue which cannot be so lightly dismissed. No workforce is exempt from mental health problems: a company with 1,000 employees can expect 200 to 300 people (as measured by standardised, structured and validated interviews) to have depression or anxiety during a year, and one suicide every decade. Each year in England, 8 million working days are lost through alcohol and drink-related disease and 80 million through other mental illness, compared with 35 million through CHD and stroke. Moreover, figures for psychiatric morbidity are likely to be minimum estimates: many people are reluctant to let their employers know that they have been depressed or otherwise mentally ill, and GPs may fail to recognise depression or to recognise that physical symptoms can be emotional in origin[3].

As a major employer, the NHS is taking action to improve the health of its own workforce. The Chief Executive has set up and is overseeing systems to test ideas for organisation of work in hospitals, which (among other benefits) are hoped to reduce absences due to mental ill-health. The mental health of NHS employees has also been selected as one of six national priorities in the NHS programme of mental health research and development, and several studies of this topic have been commissioned or are under way.

DH, in collaboration with the Confederation of British Industry (CBI) published the book *Prevention of mental ill health at work*[8], based on a conference attended by business managers, personnel officers and occupational health professionals, in September 1992. In November, DH sponsored a stand and held a Ministerial breakfast at the CBI Annual Conference to promote the strategy for health[2] and issues related to mental health in the workplace.

(vi) Services for people with severe mental illness.

A Mental Health Task Force, under the leadership of Mr David King (formerly District General Manager of Exeter Health Authority), has been established to ensure the concerted and comprehensive implementation of DH's long-standing policy to create more locally based and accessible services for the care of people with severe mental illness.

A recent follow-up study of 532 patients with schizophrenia at an interval of 3-13 years after discharge from inpatient care for an index episode[9] showed that persistent symptoms were common, but that less than 10% were inpatients when reviewed and fewer than 1% of patients or relatives sought a return to inpatient care. 90% were receiving medical or social support, with 45% under continued supervision by a psychiatrist.

Nevertheless, compliance with treatment remains a concern[10] and the Secretary of State for Health initiated further consideration of ways to assist compliance. Early intervention[11] and skills training in illness self-management[12] also have a part to play. Community psychiatric nurses can be especially effective in ensuring the delivery of psychosocial interventions[13], but there is evidence that such nurses are spending less time working with people who have severe mental illness than they would have been 10 years ago[14]. The review of mental health nursing, which started in 1992 and is chaired by Professor Butterworth, will examine the workload and most effective use of community psychiatric nurses.

(vii) Services for mentally disordered offenders

Last year's Report[15] referred to the establishment of a joint Home Office/DH review of health and social services for mentally disordered offenders and others requiring similar services. This review was completed in July and a final summary report[16] was published in November 1992. Reports from the advisory groups on finance, staffing and training; academic development and research;

people with special needs; and service needs in the community, hospital and prison; and an overview from the steering committee will be published early in 1993. Reports on learning disabilities and autism[17] and on racial and cultural issues[18] were issued for consultation in November 1992: the responses overwhelmingly supported the proposed direction of development. Two further advisory groups have now been established to look at high-security psychiatric care and psychopathic disorder.

The final summary report contains 276 recommendations: many of these relate to good practice and co-operation between agencies, and others to proposed service developments. The report emphasises that changes cannot be achieved overnight, but notes many areas in which significant progress has already been made. Following the publication of the Home Office Circular[19] which preceded the review, a number of court diversion and similar schemes, which seek to enable a mentally disordered offender to receive care and treatment outside the criminal justice system, were established through locally resourced initiatives: by June 1992, there were over 40 such schemes in England and another 30 were planned. However, only a minority of NHS purchasers are likely to have included diversion schemes in present or future purchasing plans, and more will need to consider the inclusion of such services in their plans. The Home Office currently provides funds to support psychiatric assessment within new court diversion schemes.

In April 1992, DH asked Regional Directors of Public Health (RDsPH) to assess the need for services for mentally disordered offenders[20,21]. These assessments required consultation with all agencies involved in the management and diversion of such offenders from the criminal justice system, including special hospitals, DHAs, FHSAs, GP fundholders, local authority social services and housing departments, prisons, probation services, courts, police and relevant voluntary organisations. Such assessment of need is to become a regular joint agency activity which will keep under review the whole range of services for 'difficult to place' and offender patients: this process will not only enhance a planned, co-ordinated multi-agency approach but will encourage a local responsibility for special hospital and medium-secure unit patients, and a change of emphasis from national targets for secure psychiatric provision to an approach based on local population needs[2,22,23,24].

References

1. Department of Health. *The care programme approach for people with a mental illness referred to the special psychiatrist services.* London: Department of Health, 1990 (Health Circular: HC(90)23/LASSL(90)11).
2. Department of Health. *The Health of the Nation: a strategy for health in England.* London: HMSO, 1992 (Cm. 1986).
3. Goldberg D, Huxley P. *Common Mental Disorders: a bio-social model.* London: Routledge, 1992.
4. Jenkins R. Developments in the primary care of mental illness: a look forward. *Int Rev Psychiatry.* 1992; **4**: 237-42.
5. Paykel ES, Priest RG. Recognition and management of depression in general practice: consensus statement. *BMJ* 1992; **305**: 1198-202.
6. Corney R, Jenkins R. *Counselling in general practice.* London: Routledge, 1992.
7. Jenkins R, Field V, Young R, eds. *Primary care of schizophrenia: a conference organised by Research and Development for Psychiatry and the Department of Health.* London: HMSO, 1992.
8. Jenkins R, Coney N. *Prevention of mental ill health at work.* London: HMSO, 1992.
9. Johnstone EC, ed. The disabilities and circumstances of schizophrenic patients - a follow up study. *Br J*

Psychiatry 1991: **159** (suppl 13).

10. Buchanan A. A two-year prospective study of treatment compliance in patients with schizophrenia. *Psychol Med* 1992; **22:** 787-97.

11. Birchwood M, Shepherd G. Controversies and growing points in cognitive-behavioral interventions for people with schizophrenia. *Behav Psychother* 1992; **20:** 305-42.

12. Eckman T, Wirshing WC, Marder SR, et al. Technique for training schizophrenic patients in illness self-management: a controlled trial. *Am J Psychiatry* 1992; **11:** 1549-55.

13. Brooker C, Tarrier N, Barrowclough E, Butterworth A, Goldberg D. Training community psychiatric nurses for psychosocial intervention. Report of a pilot study. *Br J Psychiatry* 1992: **160:** 836-44.

14. White E. *The third quinquennial survey of community psychiatric nursing services.* London (c/o Health Visitors Association, 50 Southwark Street, London SE1 1UN): Community Psychiatric Nursing Association, 1990.

15. Department of Health. *On the State of the Public Health: the annual report of the Chief Medical Officer of the Department of Health for the year 1991.* London: HMSO, 1992; 122.

16. Department of Health, Home Office. *Final Summary Report. Review of health and social services for mentally disordered offenders and others requiring similar services.* London: HMSO, 1992 (Cm. 2088).

17. Official Working Group on Services for People with Special Needs. *Review of health and social services for mentally disordered offenders and others requiring similar services: people with learning disabilities (mental handicap) or autism.* London: Department of Health, 1992.

18. Department of Health, Home Office. *Review of health and social services for mentally disordered offenders and others requiring similar services: services for people from black and ethnic minority groups: issues of race and culture: a discussion paper.* London: Department of Health, 1992.

19. Department of Health. *Home Office circular on provision for mentally disordered offenders.* London: Department of Health, 1990 (Executive Letter: EL (90) 168, Home Office Circular no. 66/90).

20. Department of Health. *Assessment of needs for services for mentally disordered offenders and patients with similar needs.* London: Department of Health, 1992 (Executive Letter: EL(92)24).

21. Jones D, Dean N. Assessment of need for services for mentally disordered offenders and patients with similar needs. *Health Trends* 1992; **24:** 48.

22. O'Grady J, Courtney P, Cunnane J. The provision of secure psychiatric services in Leeds; paper i. a point prevalence study. *Health Trends* 1992; **24:** 49-51.

23. Courtney P, O'Grady J, Cunnane J. The provision of secure psychiatric services in Leeds; paper ii. a survey of unmet need. *Health Trends* 1992; **24:** 51-3.

24. Department of Health. *Progress on care of mentally disordered offenders made through better service co-ordination, says Tim Yeo.* London: Department of Health, 1992 (Press Release H92/420).

(g)   Maternity and child health services

(i)   *Health Select Committee Reports on maternity services*

During 1991 and the early part of 1992, the Health Select Committee conducted an enquiry into maternity services. Its first report[1], *Maternity Services: Preconception*, was published in October 1991. The Committee's view was that preconception care is predominantly good health education and promotion. Nevertheless, it considered that improvements in the outcome of pregnancy could not be achieved by these means alone, but also required improvements in social conditions. The Committee's views were welcomed and endorsed in the Government's Response[2].

The Committee's second and final report[3], which focused on women's expectations of maternity services and whether they were being realised, was published in February 1992. The Committee concluded that there is a strong desire for continuity of care and carer throughout pregnancy and childbirth, and that most women regard midwives as the group best placed and equipped to provide such care. Moreover, the opportunity for women to exercise choice about the way care is provided would be greater if they were always seen as partners rather than patients, and were provided with full information about all available options and their implications. The Committee questioned the policy of encouraging all women to give birth in hospitals where emergency facilities were available, as it was not aware of any conclusive evidence that this policy enhanced safety for mothers and babies.

The Government's Response[4] pointed to the association of its policies with the continuing fall in perinatal mortality to the lowest rate ever recorded (8 per 1,000 total births in 1991). The Government believed that there were two main principles which should be followed in the provision of maternity services - the safety of care, and the need to enable women to make choices about the care they receive including, for women for whom the risk of complications is considered to be low, the choice of care in a low-technology environment. Several actions were planned to develop the service in line with these principles. First and foremost, an Expert Maternity Group would review care during childbirth and make recommendations: this Group began its review in 1992, and its recommendations are likely to be published for consultation in the Summer of 1993. Other initiatives included a Management Executive Task Force to produce guidance on good practice and a DH/NHS study team to examine good practice in the provision of maternity care in units led by GPs or midwives. The study team's report will be published in January 1993.

(ii) Family planning services

The Report[5] for 1991 drew attention to the continued rise in the conception rate among women aged 13-15 years; the rate in 1990 was 10.1 per 1,000. Unintended pregnancies were also common in older teenagers and associated with a high abortion rate of 22.5 per 1,000 in 1992 for women aged 16-19 years; this rate, based on provisional data, is not far short of that for women aged 20-24 years (26.2 per 1,000), which is the highest rate for any age-group.

The importance of seeking to prevent these personal tragedies was recognised in the strategy for health[6], in which family planning was identified within the theme of HIV/AIDS and sexual health as a key area for health promotion activity. The White Paper pointed to the need to develop education about sexual matters and to take steps to improve family planning services. It set a target to reduce by at least 50% the rate of conceptions among girls under 16 years-of-age by the year 2000, equivalent to no more than 4.8 per 1,000 women aged 13-15 years.

After publication of the strategy for health[6], DH set up NHS-led focus groups for each of the five key areas. The recommendations of these groups, *First Steps for the NHS*[7], were published in November 1992. With the energetic assistance of many practising professionals, DH has prepared a series of key area handbooks for publication early in 1993. The handbook on HIV/AIDS and sexual health will give particular emphasis to the importance of alliances between organisations with an involvement or interest in the development of sex education, and will set out numerous examples of local achievements. Improvement of counselling and contraception services for young people will require special sensitivity to the insecurity which is often a feature of the teenage years, and the handbook will recommend that information about these services is made much more readily available.

The Family Planning Association (FPA) and the Brook Advisory Centres continued to provide very important contributions in this area. The FPA's information service, funded by DH, is much valued by those working in family planning and related fields. During 1992, the FPA published three booklets, the *Growing Up* series[8], aimed at parents and children, and the Brook Advisory Centres issued a series of three leaflets for young people that described safer sex practices. Both organisations co-operated with Thames Television over the writing of a sex education leaflet, which was funded by DH and published in association with the drama *A Small Dance*, broadcast in June 1992. They also assisted BBC Television with the production of its *What Shall We Tell The Children* series, which is to be broadcast early in 1993.

The Report[1] for 1991 referred to DH's request to RHAs to review the provision of family planning services. These reviews were completed in 1992, and served to highlight examples of good practice but also weaknesses - particularly in the provision of counselling and contraceptive services especially designed for the young, and in the availability of emergency contraception. These analyses of services and the needs of local populations should help Regions to develop local strategies, assisted by the key area handbook. Health authorities are increasingly turning to Brook Advisory Centres for help in the provision of services for young people, and the FPA has done much useful work on the training and resource needs of doctors and nurses in primary health care teams.

Research continues to develop improved contraceptives and a wider choice of methods. Of note in 1992 was the marketing of a female condom which has been welcomed by some women. However, further studies of its efficacy are needed, particularly because the product incorporated a spermicide in trials[9] but is now sold without one.

(iii) Cervical cancer screening

Cancer is one of five key areas within the strategy for health[6]. For cervical cancer, the target is to reduce the incidence of invasive cancer by at least 20% by the year 2000. Guidance on steps to achieve this target will be included in the key area handbook on cancers, which will be published early in 1993. There has been excellent progress towards the achievement of high levels of coverage in the national cervical cancer screening programme (see Figure 5.1); if these efforts continue and due attention is paid to quality control of all aspects of the programme, this challenging target should be met.

In 1991, the National Audit Office began a study of cervical and breast cancer screening in England. Its Report[10] was published in 1992 and was scrutinised by the Public Accounts Committee[11]. The good progress made with implementation of computerised call and recall was noted. However, because the screening programme involved so many parts of the NHS, it was recognised that purchasers of services would find it challenging to draw up contracts to cover the programme. The role of the National Co-ordinating Network, which was described in the Report for 1991[12], is therefore of even greater importance than

Figure 5.1: *Screening for cervical cancer: coverage for women aged 20-64 years by District, England, 1991/92*

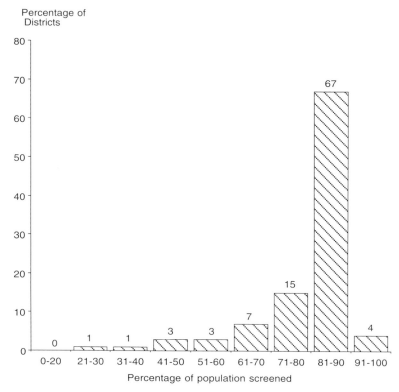

Percentage of Districts

Percentage of population screened

Source: Form KC53

before. The National Co-ordinating Network has published valuable guidelines on fail-safe actions when a smear is abnormal[13] and on clinical practice and programme management[14].

(iv) *The Human Fertilisation and Embryology (Disclosure of Information) Act 1992*

The Human Fertilisation and Embryology Act 1990[15] established the Human Fertilisation and Embryology Authority, the functions of which include the licensing and control of centres that provide treatment involving in-vitro fertilisation or the use of donated gametes. The Authority soon drew attention to difficulties for doctors and patients arising from restrictions on the disclosure of information imposed by Section 33(5) of this Act.

As a result, the Government introduced an amending Bill, the Human Fertilisation and Embryology (Disclosure of Information) Bill, which received Royal Assent on 16 July 1992[16]. The new Act permits the disclosure of information by a licensed clinician with the consent of the person to whom the information relates. Disclosure can be made without consent in connection with legal and other proceedings (including complaints) and in an emergency where there is an imminent danger to the patient's health.

(v) *Confidential Enquiry into Stillbirths and Deaths in Infancy*

As anticipated in last year's Report[17], the National Advisory Body was established early in 1992 to steer the Confidential Enquiry into Stillbirths and Deaths in Infancy (CESDI). Members were appointed in a personal capacity to reflect the range of experience and expertise needed for the enquiry. Chaired by Lady Littler, and with the assistance of a Secretariat funded by DH, the National Advisory Body prepared advice and guidance for the enquiry, which will cover England, Wales and Northern Ireland.

The CESDI programme for 1993 will comprise:

- the establishment of a prompt and comprehensive reporting scheme, to collect a minimum uniform set of information on each death, (approximately 11,000 annually in England, Wales and Northern Ireland). Standard report forms were issued at the end of 1992 for data collection to begin on 1 January 1993;

- confidential enquiries, with Regional panels of expert assessors, on 7% of the deaths - especially on babies with a birthweight of at least 2.5 kg who die during or shortly after labour;

- the setting up of case-control studies and confidential enquiries into sudden unexpected infant deaths in two Regions (Yorkshire and South Western) from February 1993, which will help to identify aspects suitable for confidential enquiry methods in the future; *and*

- dissemination and audit of guidelines on good pathology practice for necropsy examinations to support the National Advisory Body's recommendation that the information collected on CESDI cases should include post-mortem reports.

An Executive Letter issued in September 1992 gave details of the programme and the role of co-ordinators[18], and further practical advice and guidance was distributed in November. As in other forms of audit, confidential enquiries will be directed at health service interventions in an attempt to identify changes which should reduce mortality or morbidity. The National Advisory Body will review the number of cases and the categories of death that will be subject to confidential enquiries in future years.

CESDI is the first national confidential enquiry to be organised with a Regional structure. Regions were encouraged to incorporate CESDI into existing surveys, but the importance of a consistent approach to allow Regional data and results to be collated and analysed at a national level was also emphasised. DH allocated funding for Regional co-ordinators and during 1993 will provide additional funding for confidential enquiries and the evaluation of a range of pathology investigations. Some parents may refuse a necropsy because of misunderstandings about its nature, purpose and value. The National Advisory Body has therefore prepared an information leaflet for parents, to help their discussions with professional staff after a baby's death. The leaflet will be distributed early in 1993.

In the Report for 1991[17], the aim of starting data collection in 1993 was felt to be ambitious. Nevertheless, the necessary mechanisms and guidance have been put in place and the first results will be reported to Ministers in 1994.

(vi) Sudden infant death syndrome

As described in last year's Report[19], a group of experts, which had been set up by the Chief Medical Officer, advised that the risk of sudden infant death syndrome (SIDS) could be reduced if babies were not placed prone when laid down to sleep. The group's initial advice on the sleeping position of infants and cot death was widely disseminated and reinforced by the national campaign *Back to Sleep*.

During 1992, the group prepared a fuller account of the evidence for its advice, and also considered other factors for which associations with cot death have been suggested and which might also be amenable to intervention - such as cigarette smoking, the thermal environment of infants, and breast-feeding. The group also examined the need for adequate assessment of the effectiveness of the national campaign, of other changes in infant care, and of important inadvertent consequences other than the predicted fall in the incidence of cot death. Its extended report will be published during 1993.

There is now evidence to show that the risks of cot death can be reduced by a number of simple precautions on the part of those who are entrusted with the care of babies and infants, and a reduction in the prevalence of sleeping on the front has been accompanied by a striking fall in the incidence of cot death[20,21,22,23]. These studies did not, however, allow conclusions to be drawn about possible relations between cot death and changes in exposure to smoking during or after pregnancy, or changes in the thermal environment of infants.

The incidence of post-neonatal deaths attributed to SIDS in England and Wales in the years preceding and the year following the national campaign is shown in Figure 5.2. The quarterly figures for SIDS (International Classification of Diseases 9 [ICD9] 798.0) are shown in Table 5.1 which gives numbers of deaths in children aged 28 days and over. Although the incidence of cot death had been falling for the 3 years preceding the national campaign, the subsequent fall has been significantly greater.

Figure 5.2: *Post-neonatal deaths attributed to sudden infant death syndrome, England and Wales, 1986-92*

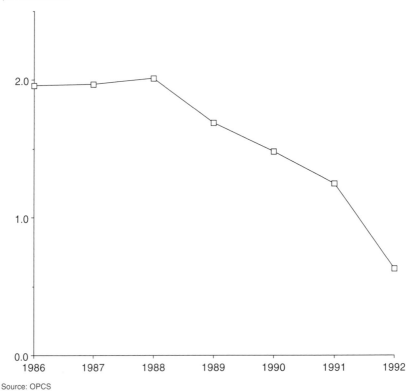

Source: OPCS

Table 5.1: *Deaths due to sudden infant death syndrome*, England and Wales, 1989-92*

Quarter	1989	1990	1991	1992
March	406	365	321	128
June	238	255	252	111
September	192	176	150	87
December	354	283	189	130

* Deaths at 28 days and over.

Source: OPCS

(vii) Prophylaxis against vitamin K deficiency bleeding in infants

By comparison with older children, newborn babies are deficient in vitamin K. In a small number of babies this deficiency is associated with bleeding without warning, which can lead to permanent disability or death. Understandably, it has been usual practice to give newborn babies prophylactic vitamin K, either intramuscularly or orally.

During 1992, a possible association between vitamin K given intramuscularly and the development of cancer in childhood was reported[24,25,26]; there was no evidence of any such association with oral vitamin K. In view of the potential importance of this report, DH asked outside experts for advice. They concluded that, although the findings could not be rebutted, the study fell far short of proving a causal association for intramuscular vitamin K, and that there was no evidence that vitamin K given orally was linked with any increased risk of childhood cancer. Further studies to resolve uncertainties about the use of intramuscular vitamin K are under way in this country and abroad.

Evidence about the use of vitamin K prophylaxis against bleeding in infants was subsequently reviewed by international experts at a meeting chaired by the President of the British Paediatric Association (BPA). They advised that the available facts did not permit a clear consensus on the safest form of prophylaxis for newborn babies, and that it would be necessary for paediatricians, midwives and other health care professionals with responsibilities in this area of practice to establish locally agreed policies for the administration of vitamin K to infants. The expert committee's report was published by the BPA[27] to assist such reviews. Almost simultaneously, the Chief Medical and Nursing Officers wrote to their colleagues to set out the background and to provide guidance on the professional issues that had been raised[28].

(viii) Review of adoption law

In July 1989, DH, other Government Departments and the Law Commission established a Working Group to review adoption law. The aim was to formulate proposals for new legislation which would reflect developments since the last review in 1972. The Working Group's report[29] was presented to Ministers in July 1992 and issued for wider consultation in October. When the responses have been analysed the Government intends, when Parliamentary time permits, to introduce new legislation.

The report emphasised that, although the number of children available for adoption has decreased, adoption as the basis of permanent transfer of a child from one family to another continues to provide an important service for children. It included 45 main recommendations on the adoption process, on the duties and responsibilities of adoption agencies, and in relation to the courts. Underpinning them is the principle that the welfare of the child is paramount, and that children have the right to be consulted about decisions concerning their adoption. Collectively the recommendations emphasised the rights of the child and the need to obtain the best outcomes for children. The report made it clear that, in the view of the Working Group, children should have the right to know that they are adopted and should have access to information about their family background - including relevant anonymised medical information.

In recognition of a continued and increasing interest in adoption across national borders, a new, more streamlined inter-country adoption process was proposed, together with new responsibilities for local authorities to provide inter-country adoption services in collaboration with voluntary adoption societies.

References

1. House of Commons. Health Committee. *Maternity Services: Preconception: fourth report from the Health Committee. Session 1990-91.* London: HMSO, 1991. Chair: Nicholas Winterton (HC 430; vol I).
2. Department of Health. *Government response to the fourth report from the Health Committee. 1990-91 session: preconception care.* London: HMSO, 1992 (Cm. 1826).
3. House of Commons. Health Committee. *Maternity Services: second report from the Health Committee. Session 1991-92.* London: HMSO, 1992. Chair: Nicholas Winterton (HC 29; vol I).
4. Department of Health. *Government response to the second report of the Health Committee. 1991-92 session: maternity services.* London: HMSO, 1992 (Cm. 2018).
5. Department of Health. *On the State of the Public Health: the annual report of the Chief Medical Officer of the Department of Health for the year 1991.* London: HMSO, 1992; 131.
6. Department of Health. *The Health of the Nation: a strategy for health in England.* London: HMSO, 1992 (Cm. 1986).
7. NHS Management Executive. *First Steps for the NHS.* Leeds: Department of Health, 1992.
8. The *Growing Up* Series. London: Family Planning Association, 1992.
9. Bounds W, Guillebaud J, Newman GB. Female condom ('Femidom'): a clinical study of its use; effectiveness and patient acceptability. *Br J Family Planning* 1992; **18**: 36-41.
10. National Audit Office. *Cervical and breast screening in England: report by the Comptroller and Auditor General.* London: HMSO, 1992 (HC 236; session 1991-92).
11. House of Commons. Committee of Public Accounts. *Cervical and Breast Screening in England: second report from the Committee of Public Accounts. Session 1992-93.* London: HMSO, 1992 (HC 58).
12. Department of Health. *On the State of the Public Health: the annual report of the Chief Medical Officer of the Department of Health for the year 1991.* London: HMSO, 1992; 134.
13. Pike C, Chamberlain J. *Guidelines on fail-safe actions.* Oxford (Oxford RHA, Old Road, Headington, Oxford OX3 7LF): National Co-ordinating Network, 1992.
14. Duncan ID. *Guidelines for clinical practice and programme management.* Oxford (Oxford RHA, Old Road, Headington, Oxford OX3 7LF): National Co-ordinating Network, 1992.
15. *Human Fertilisation and Embryology Act 1990.* London: HMS0, 1990.
16. *Human Fertilisation and Embryology (Disclosure of Information) Act 1992.* London: HMSO, 1992.
17. Department of Health. *On the State of the Public Health: the annual report of the Chief Medical Officer of the Department of Health for the year 1991.* London: HMSO, 1992; 136.
18. NHS Management Executive. *Confidential Enquiry into Stillbirths and Deaths in Infancy (CESDI).* London: Department of Health, 1992 (Executive Letter: EL(92)64).
19. Department of Health. *On the State of the Public Health: the annual report of the Chief Medical Officer of the Department of Health for the year 1991.* London: HMSO, 1992; 137.
20. Engelberts AC. *Cot death in the Netherlands: an epidemiological study.* Amsterdam: Free University Press, 1991.
21. Engelberts AC, de Jonge GA. Choice of sleeping position for infants: possible association with cot death. *Arch Dis Child* 1990; **65**: 462-7.
22. Dwyer T, Ponsonby AL, Newman NM, Gibbons LE. Prospective cohort study of prone sleeping position and sudden infant death syndrome. *Lancet* 1991; **337**: 1244-7.
23. Wigfield RE, Fleming PJ, Berry PJ, Rudd PT, Golding J. Can the fall in Avon's sudden infant death rate be explained by changes in sleeping position? *BMJ* 1992; **304**: 282-3.
24. Golding J, Birmingham K, Greenwood R, Mott M. Childhood cancer, intramuscular vitamin K, and pethidine given during labour. *BMJ* 1992; **305**: 341-6.
25. Draper GJ, Stiller CA. Intramuscular vitamin K and childhood cancer. *BMJ* 1992; **305**: 709.
26. Hull D. Vitamin K and childhood cancer. The risk of haemorrhagic disease is certain; that of cancer is not. *BMJ* 1992; **305**: 326-7.
27. British Paediatric Association. *Vitamin K Prophylaxis in Infancy. Report of an Expert Committee.* London: British Paediatric Association, 1992. Chair: Professor Sir David Hull.
28. Department of Health. *Prophylaxis against vitamin K deficiency bleeding in infants.* Heywood (Lancashire): Department of Health, 1992 (Professional letter: PL/CMO(92)20, PL/CNO(92)14).
29. Department of Health, Welsh Office. *Review of Adoption Law: Report to Ministers of an Interdepartmental Working Group.* London: Department of Health and Welsh Office, 1992. Chair: Rupert Hughes.

(h) Learning disabilities

In preparation for the implementation of new arrangements for community care in 1993, Health Service Guidelines[1], and a Local Authority Circular[2] were published in October 1992. The Health Service Guidelines[1] emphasised the responsibility of purchasers to ensure that appropriate provision is made to meet the health care needs of people with learning disabilities; reaffirmed the right of people with learning disabilities to use ordinary services with any necessary extra support; and advised purchasers to consider contracting for additional services, including specialist psychiatric assessment and treatment.

The Local Authority Circular[2] set out the direction for future developments in meeting social care needs. Services should be planned on an individual basis, parents and carers should be involved in decisions about the services to be provided, and the essential needs of disabled people should be met on a life-long basis. It described the main elements of home care, support and day services, accommodation and residential care, but did not place any specific new requirements on local authorities.

The report of the joint DH/Home Office review of services for mentally disordered offenders[3], published in 1992, identified a shortfall in services for offenders with learning disabilities (see page 122). Specific recommendations included suitable provision for people with learning disabilities, based on assessment of need, as an aim of the medium secure programme.

The inauguration in Brussels of the European Decade of Brain Research, in September 1992, will hopefully contribute to our understanding of learning disability and to the study of Down's syndrome, autism, epilepsy and other conditions which either cause or complicate any associated brain dysfunction.

References

1. Department of Health. *Health services for people with learning disabilities (mental handicap).* Heywood (Lancashire): Department of Health, 1992 (Health Service Guidelines: HSG(92)42).
2. Department of Health. *Social care for adults with learning disabilities (mental handicap).* Heywood (Lancashire): Department of Health, 1992 (Local Authority Circular: LAC(92)15).
3. Official Working Group on Services for People with Special Needs. *Review of services for mentally disordered offenders and others requiring similar services: people with learning disabilities (mental handicap) or with autism.* London: Department of Health/Home Office, 1992.

(i)   Disability and rehabilitation

During 1992, there were further developments in the field of disability and rehabilitation. At the beginning of the year, and in the wake of the publication of *Screening Children's Hearing*[1] at the end of 1991, DH hosted a multidisciplinary conference about screening children for impaired hearing.

In January, DH announced that 12 sites around the country had been selected to take part in an initiative to improve NHS rehabilitation services for people who had suffered brain injury. A research team from the University of Warwick was commissioned to manage and to evaluate the project.

In June, the National Audit Office published the report *Health services for physically disabled people aged 16 to 64*[1], which focused on identification of the needs of disabled people and their carers, and went on to examine the extent to which those needs were being met. It found that while there were still gaps in services, and also scope for more effective delivery, DH and health authorities had made great efforts to improve these services.

Also in June, a conference on 'Disability, Teamwork and Independence' was held at the King's Fund Centre. Planned by the RCGP in conjunction with DH, the conference served to increase awareness and understanding of the viewpoints of disabled people, and to discuss aspects of assessment, intervention, inter-professional collaboration and means to increase independence.

Although rehabilitation was not chosen as one of the five key areas of the strategy for health, it was identified as a strong candidate for key area status after further development and research.

The number of doctors working in the specialty of rehabilitation medicine continued to increase during 1992. A survey by the British Society of Rehabilitation Medicine identified 63 whole-time-equivalent consultant posts in the specialty, and 17 established senior registrar posts. At a Joint Planning Advisory Committee review of the specialty, a national target of 46 senior registrars was agreed.

References

1. Haggard M, Hughes E. *Screening children's hearing: a review of the literature and the implications of otitis media.* London: HMSO, 1991.
2. National Audit Office. *Health services for physically disabled people aged 16 to 64.* London: HMSO, 1992 (HC 65; session 1992-93).

(j) Prison health care

The Prison Service is committed to the concept of 'healthy prisons', as outlined in the strategy for health[1], and therefore to an increased emphasis on health promotion programmes for prisoners. Signalling this commitment, the former Prison Medical Service was relaunched in May 1992 as the Health Care Service for Prisoners. The Directorate of Health Care and the Health Advisory Committee, chaired by Sir Donald Acheson, are reviewing ways to promote prisoners' health and standards of care. Health promotion also features in a Working Party report on education and training for prison doctors, which was submitted to the Chief Medical Officer in 1992 by the Royal Colleges of Psychiatrists, General Practitioners, and Physicians, and will be published during 1993. Within the prison service, it is accepted that health promotion is a shared responsibility that requires the commitment not only of health professionals, but also education, physical education and catering staff, as well as close links with the NHS and the Health Education Authority. All of these groups are working together to devise a strategy and performance indicators for healthy prisons; these should also be published in 1993.

In the wake of the 1990 Efficiency Scrutiny[2], the Health Care Service for Prisoners is seeking closer alignment with the standards and practices of the NHS, and will become primarily a purchaser of services through contracts with the NHS and other providers. The aim is to introduce the first pilot projects in 1993, with contracts for services in mental health, primary care and genito-urinary medicine.

Each prison now has a suicide prevention management group, which aims to reduce the risk of suicide and self harm by various improvements, including the elimination of seclusion and encouragement of a therapeutic approach involving non-medical staff and voluntary agencies. The involvement of co-opted local consultant psychiatrists is also encouraged. An indication of increasingly successful liaison between prison medical officers, the Home Office and consultant psychiatrists and their teams has been the steady growth in recent years of transfers from prisons to hospital under Sections 47 and 48 of the Mental Health Act 1983[3]. In 1990 there were 325 such transfers; in 1991, 450; and during 1992 the figure rose to 611.

DH has funded an NHS liaison team project based at Brixton prison to develop and evaluate management of mentally disordered offenders. Initiatives by the Prison Service have resulted in remands to Brixton prison being considerably reduced; these are now spread amongst five prisons, enabling liaison with local psychiatric teams - a key factor to ensure the successful identification and diversion of mentally disordered offenders.

References

1. Department of Health. *The Health of the Nation: a strategy for health in England.* London: HMSO, 1992 (Cm. 1986).
2. Home Office. *Report of an efficiency scrutiny of the Prison Medical Service.* London: Home Office, 1990.
3. *Mental Health Act 1983.* London: HMSO, 1983.

(k) The health of people in later life

Demography

Over the past 150 years, average life expectancy at birth has risen from 40 to over 70 years. Most of this increase occurred in the first half of this century as a result of more effective control of infectious diseases and improvements in sanitation and nutrition. Since the 1950s, there has been further improvement in life expectancy among older age-groups: the number of people aged 65 years and above is expected to increase by 42% over the next 35 years, with an expected increase of 99% in the population aged 85 years and over. The average life expectancy at birth in England is now estimated to be 73.8 years for males and 79.2 years for females.

As mentioned in the 1990 Report[1], old age is associated with an increasing prevalence of long-standing illness and disability. During 1992 these issues were brought sharply into focus with the publication of the strategy for health[2], and an epidemiological overview[3] and a companion paper[4] setting out the current health status of older people, based on the proceedings of a DH workshop held in 1991[5].

Hospital services

Since the foundation of the NHS, the care of older people has changed dramatically, with a move away from institutional towards community-based care. Older people want to stay in their own homes for as long as possible and services have had to adapt to provide domiciliary care to a group who traditionally would have been in long-stay beds in hospital or, if less frail, in residential homes. Hospital services for elderly people have moved from chronic sick wards or isolated sanatoriums or asylums to wards in acute hospitals where older people can have access to all the facilities of a modern hospital. The value of rehabilitation to help older people return home after hospital intervention has been recognised.

Geriatricians have developed the acute services they provide to patients, admitting old people directly from Accident and Emergency Departments and GP referrals. Although there have been no randomised controlled studies of these changes, shortened lengths of hospital stay and increased numbers of discharged patients indicate an improved service to elderly people[6].

A long-standing assumption that older people are not as responsive to treatment has been disproved by research and by clinical practice. For example, older people respond as well as younger ones to treatment with thrombolytic agents for coronary artery disease, hip prostheses, antidepressants, antihypertensive therapy and many forms of surgery for cancer. Gone are the myths that one is 'old' at 65 years-of-age, or any other particular age, and that intensive treatment is a waste of time because so many symptoms are attributable to old age. The greatest changes that occur with age are multiple illness, occult presentation of disease and the association of disease with other social and environmental problems.

Types of service

Physical health

Three types of admitting service have developed: age-related, needs-related and integrated services. An age-related service admits all people over a certain age, such as 65 or more usually 75 years, to wards devoted to the care of older people. In a needs-related service, elderly people with multiple problems who are thought likely to benefit from multidisciplinary care are admitted to such wards. An integrated service admits acutely ill older people to acute medical wards for all adult age-groups, and only those who require further rehabilitation are transferred to specialist wards. Some departments have developed day hospitals to offer rehabilitation and treatment without admission so that old people can continue to live at home despite disability or chronic ill health. There are now approximately 500 consultants in the specialty, most of whom run a mixture of acute, rehabilitation and long-stay facilities as well as day hospitals.

Mental health

The past 30 years have seen a parallel development in the specialty of psychiatry of old age. Starting with a handful of specialists in the 1960s, there are now about 250 consultants who provide a comprehensive service for people aged over 65 years who have any type of psychiatric disorder. They too have moved away from an asylum or institutional-based practice to a preventive and rehabilitation-oriented approach. Most assessments take place in the patient's own home: again, the main goal is to allow older people to live in their own homes for as long as is safe and practicable.

Community and primary care

This more active approach to the care of elderly people in hospitals is mirrored in the community. DH has shown its commitment to health promotion by ensuring that GPs offer an annual check-up with particular regard to the ability to carry out every-day tasks to all those aged over 75 years. Surveillance of this type should, for example, enable the early detection of early memory loss, and allow appropriate referral to a specialist hospital medical team; early detection of cognitive impairment may ensure that reversible dementias are treated. It should also enable the GP to detect reversible or treatable causes of disability, and allow the identification of elderly people with depression who will benefit from treatment.

Health promotion

The strategy for health[2] has set out ambitious targets in the key areas of CHD and stroke, cancer, mental illness, HIV/AIDS and sexual health, and accidents. Many of these targets have relevance to elderly people, and changed lifestyle habits can confer protection to elderly people as readily as to younger age-groups. It is never too late to stop smoking cigarettes or to lose excess weight, and appropriate levels of exercise help to prevent CHD and other disorders associated with later life, such as osteoporosis.

Accidents are a major cause of ill health and death among elderly people: 70% of all fatal home accidents happen to people aged over 65 years, and more than 300,000 attend Accident and Emergency Departments each year as a result of a fall. Effective reduction of the risk of accidents would have a major impact on the health and well-being of older people, and GPs may be able to identify older people at risk during routine screening, as well as those in need of early intervention and rehabilitation for physical or mental illness.

The personal and financial burden of disability is often highest in old age. The aim must be not just to add years to life but also life to years, and so to increase the years of life after 65 years-of-age that are free from disability. A global measure of outcome, Health Life Expectancy (HALE), has been developed to determine the effectiveness at various ages (eg 65, 75 and 85 years) of preventive and therapeutic interventions by health and social services. DH will be funding a study to compare HALE estimates with various other assessments of health and other data from routine screening of older people.

'Caring for People'

There are approximately 1,258,984 registered handicapped adults in England (excluding those whose sole disability is a mental disorder), of whom 840,404 are aged over 65 years. There are approximately 600,000 people aged over 60 years with dementia in England. Care for both these groups of people is often provided by relatives or carers with little professional help or support. The implementation of *Caring for People*[7] and the new responsibilities of DHAs and local authorities should mean better targeted care which takes into account a comprehensive assessment of the health and social needs of older people and their carers. Effective collaboration between health and social services should ensure the delivery of flexible services to enable people to receive the care they need and to allow them to live independently in their own homes for as long as possible.

References

1. Department of Health. *On the State of the Public Health: the annual report of the Chief Medical Officer of the Department of Health for the year 1990.* London: HMSO, 1991.
2. Department of Health. *The Health of the Nation: a strategy for health in England.* London: HMSO, 1992 (Cm. 1986).
3. Department of Health. *The Health of Elderly People: an epidemiological overview: vol I.* London: HMSO, 1992.
4. Department of Health. *The Health of Elderly People: an epidemiological overview: vol I companion papers.* London: HMSO, 1992.
5. Department of Health. *On the State of the Public Health: the annual report of the Chief Medical Officer of the Department of Health for the year 1991.* London: HMSO, 1992.
6. Audit Commission. *Lying in Wait: the use of medical beds in acute hospitals.* London: HMSO, 1992.
7. Department of Health. *Caring for People: community care in the next decade and beyond.* London: HMSO, 1989.

(l)   Health of black and ethnic minorities

Last year's Report[1] commented on some of the variations in health and disease patterns observed in black and ethnic minority communities. It highlighted the diversity of ethnic minority groups, not only in terms of their patterns of morbidity and mortality, but also in terms of lifestyles and use of health services. Some of this variation may be explained by differences in disease patterns, but the extent to which it reflects different thresholds and perceptions of illness, or the accessibility and acceptability of services, is not known.

Reference was also made to areas identified by ethnic minority communities in which action is needed to prevent discrimination in the delivery of health services. These include:

-   provision of appropriate diet, such as Halal meat or vegetarian meals;

-   respect and facilities for religious observance and access by spiritual advisers, such as imams, pandits etc;

-   the availability of women doctors for women patients;

-   the ready availability of link workers, interpreters and advocates;

-   information in ethnic minority languages; *and*

-   respect for the patient's standards of dignity and privacy, for example by the provision of long nightdresses and long-sleeved clothing.

The Report stressed that people who work in the health service must be aware of issues that might affect ethnic minority groups and should bear them in mind to ensure the provision of high-quality health care services for the whole population.

It also pointed to the need for further research to improve the understanding of ethnic minority health and the factors that influence it. Encouraging progress has been made in improving awareness of these issues and in the planning of research projects, although it will be several years before comprehensive data are available.

Demography

Since the publication of last year's Report, the first results of the 1991 Census have become available[2]. This Census is the first in Britain to include a question on ethnic group[3]. For England as whole, responses to this question indicate that 6.2% of the population come from an ethnic minority background. This figure is slightly larger than previous estimates that were based on information on country of birth in the 1981 Census, and on ethnic origin collected by the Labour Force Survey (LFS)[4]. The main difference between the Census and LFS-based estimates is largely associated with the inclusion of a write-in category 'black other' in the Census and the use of imputation for missing responses in deriving Census counts.

The Census confirms that ethnic minorities are largely concentrated in metropolitan and industrial areas (see Figure 5.3). Conversely, in many rural areas fewer than 1% of the population belong to ethnic minority groups, with the lowest proportions found in Cumbria, Northumberland, Cornwall and Somerset. The main ethnic groups identified by the Census tend to have distinctive geographical distributions[5]. Black groups are predominantly concentrated in 11 inner London boroughs (see Figure 5.4), whereas Asians are more widely dispersed (see Figure 5.5) - for example, Bangladeshis in Tower Hamlets and Indians in Leicester, some outer London boroughs, Slough and Wolverhampton. Table 5.2 shows how this pattern is reflected in the distribution of ethnic groups in each RHA and in a selection of DHAs.

The age structure of the main ethnic groups differs from that of the overall population as a result of past patterns of migration, fertility and mortality (see figure 5.6). While 9% of the total population aged under 15 years belong to a black or ethnic minority group, the comparable figure at 65 years-of-age and over is only 1% (see Figure 5.7). The proportion aged 45-64 years has now reached just over 4%, mainly comprising black Caribbeans and Indians. Over the next few years, an increasing proportion of older people will come from ethnic minority communities, and this change will have implications for the delivery of health services.

Concern has been expressed about the reporting of ethnicity in the Census[6]; the accuracy of the 1991 Census counts of ethnic groups will become clearer once results of the audit of the quality of, and coverage checks on, the Census become available towards the end of 1993.

139

Table 5.2: *Ethnic composition by Regional Health Authority and selected District Health Authorities, England, 1991*

Area	All ethnic groups		Black			Asian					All others	Total population (1991 Census count)
			Caribbean	African	Other	Indian	Pakistani	Bangladeshi	Chinese	Other Asian		
	%	Number	%	%	%	%	%	%	%	%	%	Number
England	6.19	2910865	1.05	0.44	0.37	1.75	0.96	0.34	0.30	0.40	0.58	47055204
Regional Health Authorities												
Northern	1.27	38547	0.04	0.05	0.06	0.26	0.31	0.12	0.16	0.10	0.17	3026732
Yorkshire	4.98	177869	0.43	0.10	0.21	1.04	2.28	0.20	0.17	0.17	0.37	3573894
Trent	4.42	203580	0.56	0.09	0.24	2.08	0.65	0.09	0.18	0.16	0.37	4606495
East Anglian	2.14	43403	0.25	0.12	0.35	0.32	0.29	0.08	0.18	0.18	0.37	2027784
North West Thames	16.07	562041	2.35	1.13	0.69	6.25	1.35	0.52	0.67	1.49	1.62	3497103
North East Thames	13.90	513469	2.89	1.76	0.88	2.71	1.16	1.83	0.60	0.96	1.11	3693376
South East Thames	7.72	278518	2.34	1.34	0.66	1.22	0.20	0.22	0.46	0.51	0.77	3607552
South West Thames	6.95	206645	1.34	0.64	0.41	1.58	0.59	0.18	0.42	0.93	0.87	2971851
Wessex	1.55	45020	0.17	0.07	0.13	0.37	0.07	0.11	0.19	0.14	0.31	2911833
Oxford	5.12	127775	0.82	0.19	0.34	1.38	1.10	0.14	0.27	0.33	0.56	2494128
South Western	1.39	44778	0.31	0.06	0.15	0.24	0.10	0.05	0.14	0.09	0.26	3219872
West Midlands	8.24	424359	1.52	0.10	0.37	3.08	1.91	0.38	0.19	0.22	0.47	5150246
Mersey	1.49	35281	0.12	0.14	0.22	0.19	0.07	0.05	0.31	0.09	0.31	2360258
North Western	5.35	209580	0.48	0.15	0.28	1.30	1.93	0.35	0.26	0.17	0.43	3914080
District Health Authorities with the largest percentage of population belonging to ethnic groups												
Newham	42.31	89767	7.19	5.59	1.58	13.03	5.89	3.84	0.81	2.97	1.40	212170
West Birmingham	40.24	81730	11.20	0.52	1.62	14.36	6.72	2.92	0.48	1.01	1.41	203082
District Health Authorities with the smallest percentage of population belonging to ethnic groups												
North West Durham	0.37	320	0.01	0.02	0.02	0.14	0.02	0.02	0.05	0.02	0.05	86046
West Cumbria	0.36	493	0.02	0.01	0.05	0.05	0.02	0.01	0.08	0.04	0.08	136596

Source: OPCS 1991 Census

Figure 5.3: *Percentage of total population that is of ethnic minority origin by County district, England and Wales, 1991*
Greater Manchester

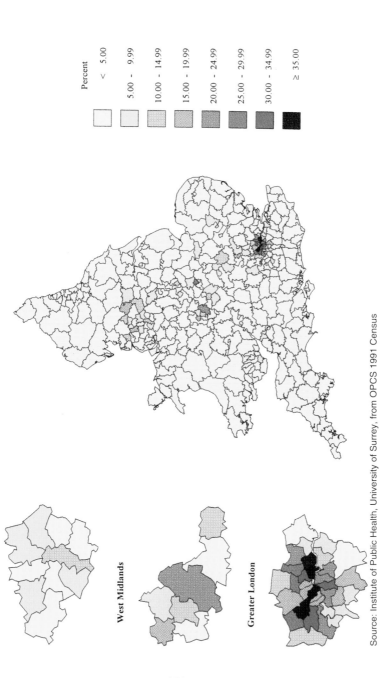

Percent

< 5.00

5.00 - 9.99

10.00 - 14.99

15.00 - 19.99

20.00 - 24.99

25.00 - 29.99

30.00 - 34.99

≥ 35.00

West Midlands

Greater London

Source: Institute of Public Health, University of Surrey, from OPCS 1991 Census

Figure 5.4: *Percentage of total population that is of 'black' ethnic origin by County district, England and Wales, 1991*

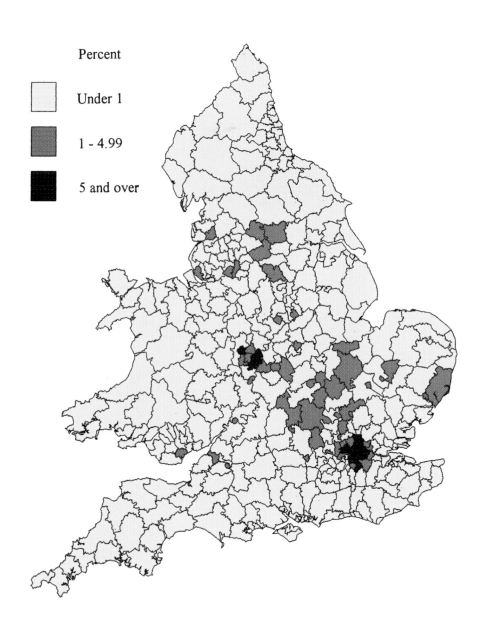

Source: Institute of Public Health, University of Surrey, from OPCS 1991 Census

Figure 5.5: *Percentage of total population that is of 'Asian' ethnic origin* by County district, England and Wales, 1991*

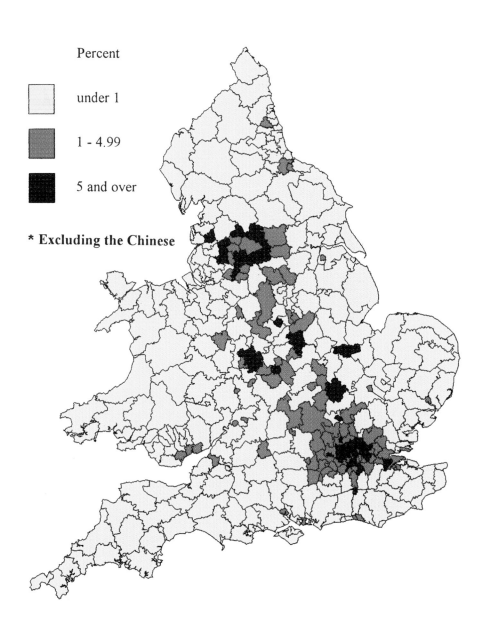

Percent

under 1

1 - 4.99

5 and over

* Excluding the Chinese

* Excludes those of Chinese origin.

Source: Institute of Public Health, University of Surrey, from OPCS 1991 Census

Figure 5.6: *Age distribution of white population and of all ethnic groups, England, 1991*

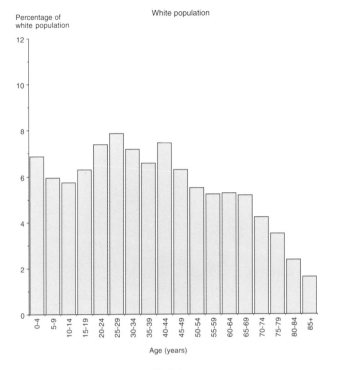

White population

Percentage of
white population

Age (years)

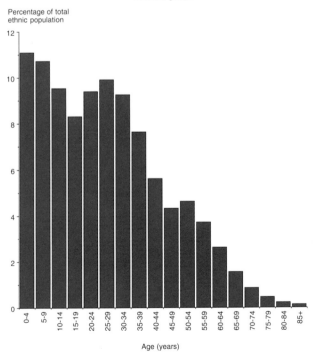

All ethnic groups

Percentage of total
ethnic population

Age (years)

Source: OPCS 1991 Census

Figure 5.7: *Percentage of the population belonging to ethnic minority groups by age, England, 1991*

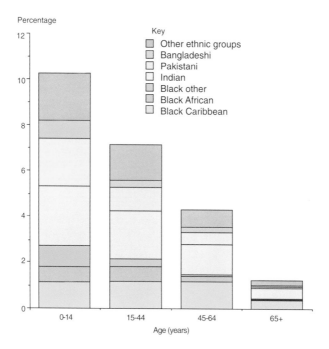

Note: The remaining percentage of the population is white.

Source: OPCS 1991 Census

Action to improve the health of ethnic minority groups

Much of DH's work as described elsewhere in this Report will affect the health of people in ethnic minority groups. Implementation of the strategy for health[7], for example, must take account of the particular circumstances of people from ethnic minorities; otherwise, in those Districts where they are most numerous, the targets will not be met. Within this framework of general policies, several initiatives have been specifically targeted towards ethnic minority communities, either to improve access to, or the quality of, available health services.

Information and education

DH supported the production of a wide range of educational material that covered various issues and was intended to benefit many minority groups (see Table 5.3). Some initiatives are targeted at specific communities or groups (such as the videos describing mental health services), while others were intended for training professional staff about particular requirements, such as the child care needs of Afro-Caribbean and Asian communities. Much of this activity has been in response to requests from the communities or health professionals themselves - such as the video on menopause, produced in response to a need identified by the Asian Women's Conference. The *Patient's Charter*[8] was translated into 11 different languages so that ethnic minorities have information about the quality of service they should expect.

145

Table 5.3: *Information and educational material supported by Department of Health, 1992*

Topic	Information
Menopause	Video produced by UK Asian Women's Conference, available in Hindi, Urdu, Gujerati, Bengali, and Punjabi.
Stress and stress management	Video and support materials produced by Health Promotion Unit, Coventry, for Asian women in Bengali, Gujerati, Hindi, Urdu, Punjabi and English.
Child protection and female genital mutilation	Video and supporting material produced by Foundation for Women's Health Research and Development (FORWARD).
Managing your asthma	Video produced by National Asthma Campaign for the Asian community in Hindi, Urdu, Gujerati, Bengali and Punjabi.
Mental health	Video produced by the Maudsley Outreach and Treatment Team (MOST) to highlight available mental health services, available in Punjabi, Bengali, Turkish, Vietnamese, Cantonese, Afro-Caribbean dialect and English.
Child care	Video produced by Voluntary Organisations Liaison Council for Under Fives (VOLCUF) to describe child care needs of Afro-Caribbean and Asian communities.
Diabetes mellitus	Video produced by British Diabetic Association to explain living with diabetes, available in five Asian languages.
A health pack for women	A set of leaflets produced by Bolton Health Authority and Ealing Health Authority (commissioned by the Health Education Authority) about health issues for Asian women, available in Hindi, Gujerati, and Urdu.

DH also supported several conferences which highlighted ethnic minority health issues, including a conference at the Royal College of Physicians to assess the needs of ethnic minority communities and a major European conference held in London in November 1992, which focused on the challenge of conveying information about HIV and AIDS to the Asian population.

Support of NHS functions

Work continued on the collection of ethnicity data within the NHS. DH commissioned the King's Fund Centre to develop approaches to community consultation with ethnic minority communities so that the NHS could more effectively deliver health care based on identified need; a report is expected in

1993. The Office of Public Management was also funded to develop ways to set priorities and to identify processes that lead to effective purchasing of health care for ethnic minority groups.

Home accident prevention

Last year's Report[1] identified the need for more research on this topic, and accidents were identified as a key area in the strategy for health[7]. Since 1990, DH and the Department of Trade and Industry have funded the Royal Society for the Prevention of Accidents to look at the promotion of home safety among Asian, Chinese and Vietnamese communities. This study was completed in 1992 and preliminary results indicate that the home safety needs expressed by the minority communities studied were similar to those of the white population, but that there are striking differences in the way that messages about home safety should be delivered. The full report is expected in 1993.

Haemoglobinopathy services

During 1992, the NHS Management Executive asked Regions to include genetics services among services which needed to be kept under review[9]. This review will be of particular interest to people from ethnic minorities because it covers the screening services for sickle cell disorder and thalassaemia. The Standing Medical Advisory Committee Working Party on sickle cell disorder and thalassaemia continued its work and will report in 1993.

Mental health

As noted in last year's Report[1], rates of mental illness differ between ethnic groups: the incidence of schizophrenia appears to be several times higher among black Caribbean people in England compared with those living in Jamaica. Misdiagnosis, genetic, viral or obstetric factors, social adversity and racism have been advanced as possible explanations: one study has shown that black African and Caribbean patients are less likely than white British patients to receive a diagnosis of anxiety or depression from their GP[10]. Although reported rates of anxiety and depression among Asian people are the same or lower than in the general population, there has been a worrying rise in the suicide rate among young Asian women[11].

There are also ethnic differences in the pathways to psychiatric care. Black African and Caribbean people with schizophrenia are less likely than non-black people to have seen their GP before hospital admission[12] and are more likely to be compulsorily detained in hospital under the Mental Health Act 1983[13] and to receive depot medication[14].

DH has funded projects to improve understanding of ethnic minority mental health, including a prospective study of severe mental illness among black and white populations to assess the long-term outcome of psychosis. Grants have also been made to *Nafsiyat* (a charitable intercultural therapy centre), the

Maudsley Outreach and Support Team, and the Confederation of Indian Organisations. Two King's Fund initiatives to take forward new models for meeting the mental health needs of black and ethnic communities are under way.

Usage and abusage

The rise in interest in the health of people who are from ethnic minority communities has led to a substantial increase in the quantity of health research which uses the concept of 'ethnicity' or 'race' to describe or to explain patterns of disease, use of health services and effectiveness of treatments[14]. However, it is vital that there is a shared understanding of the concepts and terms used. Clear distinctions between some people might be possible in terms of phenotypical features, or 'race', but geographical variation in gene frequency is gradual and in many instances there are no sharp lines of demarcation by means of easily identifiable racial characteristics. Over the last 20 years or so, the use of 'race' has been largely replaced by the term ethnicity - which refers more to shared cultural characteristics and national identity. Again the lines of demarcation may be blurred, but (in contrast to race) ethnicity is usually identified from within the groups, and identification with such a group is made by individuals rather than imposed from outside.

There are some practical difficulties associated with use of the concept of ethnicity: in particular, it may vary over time according to social and political context and the definition of groupings may be inconsistent[15]. For example, the term 'Asian' is commonly used in Britain to denote people with origins in the Indian Subcontinent, yet in the United States tends to refer to people from East and South-East Asia. Similarly, a wide variety of sub-classifications might be used within the term 'Asian' - such as 'Indian', 'Asian Indian', 'South Asian', or 'predominantly Asian'[16]. Parallel examples may be found for other ethnic groupings. These difficulties with terminology have no simple solutions, and are compounded by the fact that ethnicity is self-defined and individuals may change their mind about the labels that they find acceptable to have applied to them. Researchers and others must understand the basis of these concepts and clearly identify the ethnic groups to whom they refer.

The inclusion of ethnicity within NHS data would provide a wealth of information and give an unprecedented opportunity to examine the use of health services by different ethnic groups. However, for data based on the concept of ethnicity the method of data collection and the categories used are important. The broad categories used in the 1991 Census may not be sufficiently sensitive to identify important local variations. Nevertheless, to ensure comparability, any local classification needs to aggregate back to a set of defined common categories for national comparisons. Locally collected data must not be used as a substitute for working with local ethnic minority populations regarding the accessibility and quality of services available. As with any large data set, statistically significant associations will be noted. Particular care needs to be given to the interpretation of such associations, which may not imply direct causal relations.

The way ahead

In September, the Secretary of State for Health asked Baroness Cumberlege, Parliamentary Under Secretary of State for Health in the House of Lords, to take responsibility for improvements to the NHS services received by ethnic minorities. One of Baroness Cumberlege's first actions was to hold a workshop with 13 groups from ethnic minority communities to listen to their views and experiences. A Task Force, with representatives from consumer groups, the NHS and DH, was set up to recommend action to ensure the best possible provision of health services for ethnic minorities, and is expected to report in 1993. During the year, the Secretary of State for Health chaired a Working Group on ethnic minority employment in the NHS. This group has been set up to advise her on promoting equality of opportunity for black and ethnic minority health service staff. She is expected to announce the action she intends to take in 1993.

References

1. Department of Health. *On the State of the Public Health: the Annual Report of the Chief Medical Officer of the Department of Health for the year 1991.* London: HMSO, 1992; 8-9, 54-77.
2. Office of Population Censuses and Surveys. *1991 Census: preliminary report for England and Wales.* London: HMSO, 1992.
3. Sillitoe K, White P. Ethnic group and the British Census: the search for a question. *J Roy Statistical Soc (Series A)* 1992; **155:** 2.
4. Haskey J. Ethnic minority populations resident in private households: estimates by county and metropolitan district of England and Wales. *Population Trends* 1991; **63:** 22-35.
5. Balarajan R, Raleigh VS. The ethnic populations of England and Wales: the 1991 Census. *Health Trends* 1992; **24:** 113-6.
6. Leech K. A question in dispute: the debate about an 'ethnic' question in the Census. London: Runnymede Trust, 1989.
7. Department of Health. *The Health of the Nation: a strategy for health in England.* London: HMSO, 1992 (Cm. 1986).
8. Department of Health. *The Patient's Charter.* London: Department of Health, 1991.
9. NHS Management Executive. *Monitoring issues outside corporate contracts 1992/93.* London: Department of Health, 1992 (Executive Letter: EL(92)66).
10. Lloyd K. Ethnicity: primary care and non-psychotic disorders. *Int Rev Psychiatry* 1992; **4:** 257-66.
11. Soni Raleigh V, Balarajan R. Suicide and self-burning among Indians and West Indians in England and Wales. *Br J Psychiatry* 1992; **161:** 365-8.
12. Harrison G, Holton A, Neilson D, Owens D, Boot D, Cooper J. Severe mental disorder in Afro-Caribbean patients: some social, demographic and service factors. *Psychol Med* 1989; **19:** 683-96.
13. *Mental Health Act 1983.* London: HMSO, 1983.
14. Lloyd K, Moodley P. Psychotropic medication and ethnicity: an inpatient survey. *Soc Psychiatry Psychiatr Epidemiol* 1992; **27:** 95-101.
15. Sheldon TA, Parker H. Race and ethnicity in health research. *J Publ Health Med* 1992; **14:** 104-10.
16. Bhopal RS, Phillimore P, Kohli HS. Inappropriate use of the term 'Asian': an obstacle to ethnicity and health research. *J Publ Health Med* 1991; **13:** 244-6.

CHAPTER 6

COMMUNICABLE DISEASES

(a) HIV infection and AIDS

Surveillance

Monitoring systems

One of the objectives of the strategy for health[1] is to improve arrangements for the monitoring and surveillance of HIV infection and AIDS and of other sexually transmitted diseases (see page 160). The main methods of HIV/AIDS surveillance in England are the voluntary confidential reporting systems operated by the Public Health Laboratory Service (PHLS) AIDS Centre at the Communicable Disease Surveillance Centre (CDSC)[2], and the Government's programme of anonymised HIV surveys which is implemented by CDSC[3]. More detailed information from voluntary named HIV tests at 18 laboratories is provided through a PHLS collaborative study[4]. Data on infection in children are compiled by the Institute of Child Health in collaboration with CDSC from confidential reports by paediatricians via the British Paediatric Surveillance Unit[5]; by haemophilia centre directors to the Oxford Haemophilia Centre; by obstetricians to the national study of HIV in pregnancy; and from reports directly to CDSC.

The anonymised HIV surveys have been designed to generate estimates of HIV prevalence in various population groups and to indicate trends over time. The survey methods have been developed between 1990 and 1992 under peer review through the Medical Research Council's (MRC's) Committee on Epidemiological Studies of AIDS. In addition to the Government's programme, the Institute of Child Health has organised unlinked, anonymous studies on dried blood spots from newborn infants in three of the four Thames health Regions[6].

Further insight into the HIV epidemic can be gained from studies of sexual behaviour, notably the first results from the National Study of Sexual Attitudes and Lifestyles which were published at the end of 1992[7]. Reports of other sexually transmitted diseases such as gonorrhoea and chlamydia (see page 160) are also a useful indicator of sexual behaviour in particular groups.

Progress of the epidemic in England

AIDS

1,388 cases of AIDS were reported in England in 1992. This brought the cumulative total of AIDS cases reported since 1982 to 6,433, of whom 3,942 are known to have died. Detailed breakdown of the reported cases is given in Table 6.1. As in previous years, the majority of reports have been from the Thames health Regions. Ascertainment of AIDS cases is likely to be more than 85% complete although delays of a year or more may sometimes occur between diagnosis and reporting. It is possible that those who survive longest may be subject to the greatest reporting delays, which might in turn lead to a tendency to underestimate the numbers of living patients with AIDS[8].

AIDS incidence does not reflect current HIV incidence because people newly diagnosed to have AIDS were probably infected some 10 years ago. The greatest proportional increase in AIDS cases during 1992 continued to be among people exposed to HIV through heterosexual sex (see Figure 6.1), although the absolute number remains small. Reports of AIDS in men who have had sex with men continued to rise and still dominate the reporting picture.

Figure 6.1: *AIDS cases: total numbers and numbers where infection was probably acquired through sexual intercourse between men and women, England, by*

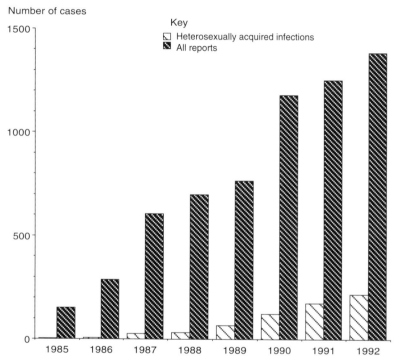

Source: CDSC

HIV infection

A further 2,294 individuals were reported to have HIV infection in England during 1992, bringing the cumulative total of such reports since 1984 to 16,768 (see Table 6.2 and Figure 6.2). However, there are many reasons why people might (or might not) seek HIV testing and these reports must be interpreted in that context. Various sources[9] indicate that unsafe sexual practices which put people at high risk of acquisition of HIV continue among homosexual men. This view is supported by data from the Government's programme of anonymised HIV surveys, which will be published at the beginning of 1993.

Table 6.1: *AIDS cases and known deaths by exposure category and date of report, England, 1982-31 December 1992*

(Numbers subject to revision as further data are received or duplicates identified)

How persons probably acquired the virus	Jan 91-Dec 91		Jan 92-Dec 92		Jan 82-Dec 92		
	Cases	Deaths	Cases	Deaths	Cases	Deaths	
	Number	Number	Number	Number	Number	Number	%
Sexual intercourse:							
between men	920	404	1010	219	5003	3126	62
between men and women							
'high risk' partner*	14	7	20	5	62	33	
other partner abroad**	132	53	166	39	482	223	47
other partner UK	17	8	17	4	51	25	
under investigation	-	-	3	2	4	3	
Injecting drug use (IDU)	51	21	50	18	202	111	55
IDU and sexual intercourse							
between men	20	11	22	6	105	69	66
Blood							
Blood factor	52	24	43	23	299	227	76
(eg haemophiliacs)							
Blood or tissue transfer							
(eg transfusion)							
Abroad	5	-	3	-	43	26	67
UK	3	2	2	-	29	22	
Mother to child	14	6	26	9	69	30	43
Other/undetermined	26	13	26	9	84	47	56
Total	1254	549	1388	334	6433	3942	61

* Men and women who had sex with injecting drug users, or with those infected through blood factor treatment or blood transfusion, and women who had sex with bisexual men.

** Includes persons without other identified risks who are from, or who have lived in, countries where the major route of HIV-1 transmission is through sexual intercourse between men and women.

Source: CDSC

Table 6.2: *HIV antibody-positive people by exposure category and date of report, England, to 31 December 1992*
(Numbers subject to revision as further data are received or duplicates identified)

How persons probably acquired the virus	Jan 91-Dec 91			Jan 92-Dec 92			Nov 84-Dec 92				
	Male	Female	NK†	Male	Female	NK†	Male	Female	NK†	Total	%
Sexual intercourse:											
between men	1498	-	-	1347	-	-	10800	-	-	10800	64
between men and women											
'high risk' partner*	13	31	-	4	36	-	46	233	-	279	2
other partner abroad**	211	208	1	232	226	-	845	744	5	1594	10
other partner UK	22	25	-	17	28	-	80	103	-	183	1
under investigation	11	8	-	23	37	-	61	72	-	133	1
Injecting drug use (IDU)	131	61	-	115	48	-	949	446	5	1400	8
IDU and sexual intercourse											
between men	23	-	-	24	-	-	233	-	-	233	1
Blood											
Blood factor (eg haemophiliacs)	3	-	-	10	-	-	1076	9	-	1085	6
Blood or tissue transfer (eg transfusion)											
Abroad/UK	7	14	-	12	7	-	74	76	1	151	1
Mother to child	17	11	-	19	14	-	70	59	-	129	1
Other/undetermined	49	22	1	73	20	2	637	106	38	781	5
Total	1985	380	2	1876	416	2	14871	1848	49	16768	100

† NK = Not known (sex not stated on report).

* Men and women who had sex with injecting drug users, or with those infected through blood factor treatment or blood transfusion, and women who had sex with bisexual men.

**Includes persons without other identified risks who are from, or who have lived in, countries where the major route of HIV-1 transmission is through sexual intercourse between men and women.

Source: CDSC

153

Figure 6.2: *HIV antibody-positive people: total numbers and numbers where infection was probably acquired through sexual intercourse between men and women, England, by year of report to 31 December 1992*

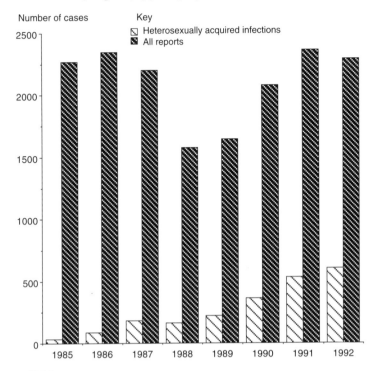

Source: CDSC

Interim results from anonymised surveys up to mid-1992 indicate a prevalence of HIV infection of about 1 in 500 among pregnant women in participating clinics in London, with a much lower prevalence outside London. This relatively high prevalence among pregnant women in London is corroborated by the findings of a small pilot survey of attenders in various clinical specialties in two London hospitals. In surveys of genito-urinary medicine (GUM) clinics, HIV infection was found in 1 in 5 homosexual men, 1 in 90 heterosexual men and 1 in 150 heterosexual women in the two participating London hospitals, compared with 1 in 20 homosexual men, 1 in 370 heterosexual men and 1 in 600 heterosexual women surveyed in clinics outside London.

Comparison of the anonymised survey results with the proportion of those tested who knew that they were seropositive indicates that a relatively large number of HIV infected people may be unaware of their infection (see Figure 6.3). This finding reinforces the need for caution in interpretation of data from voluntary HIV testing.

In December 1992, guidance was issued on additional sites for HIV antibody testing, voluntary HIV antibody testing for women attending antenatal clinics, and partner notification[10].

Figure 6.3: *Estimated proportions of HIV infections that had been diagnosed by voluntary named testing, England and Wales, 1990-92*

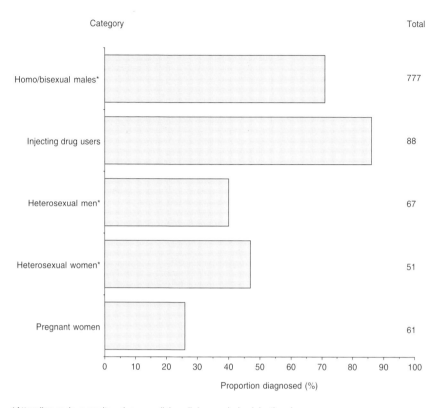

*Attending various genito-urinary medicine clinics; excludes injecting drug users.

Source: *Commun Dis Rep* **3:** R1-11

HIV in blood donations

During 1992, 2.9 million blood donations were tested with anti-HIV-1+2 combined tests. Twenty-six donations (from 15 males and 11 females) were found to be HIV-seropositive, or 1 in 111,540 (0.001%). The number of new donors tested was 349,000, of whom 13 were seropositive, ie 1 in 26,850 (0.004%). No donations were found to be anti-HIV-2-seropositive during 1992.

Table 6.3 shows the number of donations tested in the United Kingdom (UK) between the autumn of 1985 and the end of 1992, together with the number of donations confirmed as HIV-seropositive. The male/female ratio of seropositive donations in 1992 was 1.36:1. This ratio is much lower than in the past and, for the first time, there were more HIV-1-seropositive new female donors than new male donors (8 and 5, respectively) during the year. The exact numbers of male and female donors is not known, but from previous figures they are unlikely to be significantly different. In 1992, again for the first time since screening was introduced, there were no male HIV-1-seropositive donations from South East

155

England. As usual, most anti-HIV-seropositive donors were in the age-groups 21-30 and 31-40 years.

Table 6.3: *HIV in blood donations in the United Kingdom, October 1985 to December 1992*

Year	Donations tested (million)	Donations confirmed HIV-seropositive			
		Male	Female	Total	%
1985 (October-December)	0.6	13	0	13	0.002
1986	2.64	44	9	53	0.002
1987	2.59	18	5	23	0.001
1988	2.64	18	5	23	0.001
1989	2.74	25	12	37	0.001
1990	2.82	23*	12	35*	0.001
1991	2.95	20†	7	27†	0.001
1992	2.90	15	11	26	0.001
Total	19.88	176	61	237	0.001

* Includes one anti-HIV-2-seropositive donation.
† One HIV-1-seropositive male donor who gave blood during 1991 was reported after last year's Report was compiled.

Source: National Blood Transfusion Service Directorate

Donors were asked about factors that might be relevant to their HIV seropositivity. Only half have yet been interviewed, of whom 4 had engaged in homosexual activities, 4 were female partners of high-risk individuals, 1 had herself had a blood transfusion in the past, and 3 female donors were thought probably to have acquired the infection heterosexually from a partner who could not be identified as having a high-risk activity.

Progress of the epidemic world-wide

The World Health Organization (WHO) estimated that, by the end of 1992, approximately 13 million people world-wide had been infected with HIV, of whom 2.5 million had developed AIDS. WHO has further estimated that about 1 million new infections were acquired in the second half of 1992, mostly in sub-Saharan Africa and South and South East Asia.

Table 6.4 and Figure 6.4 compare the cumulative totals of AIDS cases reported in the European Community (EC) countries up to the end of 1992.

Public education

The Government's strategy on HIV and AIDS has been given renewed impetus by publication of the strategy for health[1], in which HIV/AIDS and sexual health is designated a key area for action. All aspects of HIV prevention - whether national or local, general or targeted at particular groups of the population - are now considered within the wider field of sexual health. This vital development not only maintains the high priority given to the control of HIV infection at a national level, but also recognises the complex issues that surround sexual health and ensures that full account is taken of all relevant subjects. The Health

Education Authority's (HEA's) HIV and AIDS education programmes in England and in the UK as a whole have been set within the broader context of sexual health.

Table 6.4: *AIDS cases reported to WHO by EC countries: cumulative totals at 31 December 1992*

Country	Number of cases	Cumulative cases/ million population†
Spain	17029	441
France	22939	403
Denmark	1120	215
Italy	15780	272
Netherlands	2478	163
Germany*	9205	114
Belgium	1297	130
Luxembourg	57	143
UK	6929	120
Portugal	1191	113
Ireland	308	88
Greece	721	70

* Includes the former East Germany.

† Cumulative cases per million population are now calculated directly; the population estimates used to derive these figures in previous Reports are therefore omitted from the table this year.

Source: European Centre for the Epidemiological Monitoring of AIDS

Figure 6.4: *Reported AIDS cases in Europe: cumulative rates to December 1992*

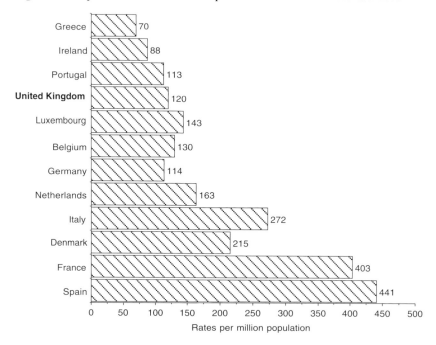

Source: European Centre for the Epidemiological Monitoring of AIDS

National initiatives

The HEA's HIV, AIDS and Sexual Health Programme includes broad-based and targeted national campaigns, and an overall strategy and operational plan have been drawn up in the light of the objectives and targets set out in the strategy for health[1].

At the beginning of 1992, a television campaign based on personal testimonies was under way, alongside a condom advertisement which had been successfully transferred from cinema to late-night television. A second cinema advertisement was moved to television during the year, also for late-night viewing but at an earlier time than had previously been permitted by broadcasting authorities. The summer campaign again highlighted risky sexual behaviour during holidays, with particular use of personal testimonies on radio, supported by cinema and press advertising. The importance of making the purchase and use of condoms a normal and acceptable fact of life and sexual activity has been a central theme of these campaigns.

Targeted advertising has been further developed for men who have sex with men; the central themes are to challenge complacency about personal risk and to emphasise the need for adopting and sustaining safer sex practices. Information 'facts cards' that deal with specific concerns have been produced for circulation in gay bars and clubs. These initiatives are aimed at any man who might have a sexual relationship with another man, not just at those who identify themselves as exclusively homosexual.

Black and ethnic minority groups

Initiatives developed in 1991 were continued, supported by a new poster campaign in the Summer of 1992 and radio advertisements in a wide range of languages. Support was given to ethnic minority groups through the system of Section 64 grants and a number of refugee and ethnic minority groups received money for specific projects from the World AIDS Day Small Grants scheme run by the Department of Health (DH).

Young people

Several advertisement campaigns have been run in magazines for young people, some aimed to encourage young women to take control of their own sexual health. The HEA funded a second Christmas pop video with a sexual health message for distribution in clubs and pubs; this was developed by Network Scotland (the Scottish managers of the National AIDS Helpline).

The Department for Education published the booklet *HIV and AIDS: a guide for the education service*[11] for distribution in secondary schools in 1991. Its up-to-date information on HIV and AIDS has helped teachers to deal with the sensitive issues involved: teaching about HIV is now mandatory within the Science Order of the National Curriculum. In December 1992, guidance on the management of children infected with HIV was issued to local authorities[12].

Local initiatives

National mass media campaigns to maintain public awareness about HIV/AIDS, and to secure behavioural changes, continue to be strengthened and supported by local initiatives. DH provides funds for local HIV prevention work by Regional and District Health Authorities, and HIV Prevention Co-ordinators have been appointed in most Districts. The HEA funded a third national conference for these District co-ordinators in November 1992, at which their role within the new structure of the National Health Service (NHS) was considered and reports were heard on longstanding projects aimed at men who have sex with men, injecting drug users, young people and members of black and ethnic minority groups. Although these local initiatives for specific communities may not immediately be visible at national level, they provide the bedrock of HIV prevention activity.

The Ministerially led AIDS Action Group completed its work in August 1992. The Action Group's findings were taken into account in the development of practical advice to be incorporated into a handbook to support the HIV/AIDS and sexual health key area of the strategy for health[1]. They will include guidance on local HIV prevention, based on work with target audiences by the six Districts represented. The Action Group pointed to a need for more intensive prevention efforts among men who have sex with men and among ethnic minority groups. The handbook and other recommendations derived from the work of the Action Group will be distributed during 1993.

The National AIDS Helpline

The National AIDS Helpline continues to support national public education initiatives by providing a permanent source of confidential advice and information about all aspects of HIV infection and AIDS. In 1992, it dealt with over 700,000 enquiries on a wide range of topics - nearly 60% of which were from young people aged 16-30 years, a key group to reach in terms of sexual health. 1992 also saw greater use of telephone services in ethnic minority languages during special HEA campaigns.

Although basic aspects of knowledge and awareness about HIV infection and AIDS still need to be addressed, the National AIDS Helpline now has to deal with increasingly sophisticated enquiries, with detailed information about HIV transmission, safer sexual practices and serological testing regularly being sought. A survey of callers who used the Helpline during 1992 was conducted by the British Market Research Bureau on behalf of the Department. Results indicate callers were overwhelmingly favourable to the service received; a high proportion would use it again if needed and would recommend it to others.

References

1. Department of Health. *The Health of the Nation: a strategy for health in England.* London: HMSO, 1992 (Cm. 1986).
2. Public Health Laboratory Service AIDS Centre. The surveillance of HIV-1 infection and AIDS in England and Wales. *Commun Dis Rep* 1991; **1**: R51-6.
3. Public Health Laboratory Service AIDS Centre et al. The unlinked anonymous HIV prevalence monitoring programme in England and Wales: preliminary results. *Commun Dis Rep* 1991; **1**: R69-76.

4. Waight PA, Rush AM, Miller E. Surveillance of HIV infection by voluntary testing in England. *Commun Dis Rep* 1992; **2:** R85-90.
5. Lynn R, Hall SM. The British Paediatric Surveillance Unit: activities and developments in 1990 and 1991. *Commun Dis Rep* 1992; **2:** R145-8.
6. Ades AE, Parker S, Cubitt D, et al. Two methods for assessing the risk factor composition of the HIV-1 epidemic in heterosexual women: South-east England, 1988-91. *AIDS* 1992; **6:** 1031-6.
7. Johnson A, Wadsworth J, Wellings K, Bradshaw S, Freed J. Sexual lifestyles and HIV risk. *Nature* 1992; **336:** 410-2.
8. Whitmore-Overton SE, Tillett HE, Evans BG, Allardice GM. Improved survival from diagnosis of AIDS in adult cases in the UK and bias due to reporting delays. *AIDS* (in press).
9. Evans BG, Mortimer JY, McGarrigle CA, et al. Continuing HIV-1 transmission among men who have sex with men in England and Wales. *BMJ* (in press).
10. Department of Health. *Department of Health Guidance: Additional sites for HIV antibody testing; offering voluntary named HIV antibody testing to women receiving antenatal care; partner notification for HIV infection.* London: Department of Health, 1992 (Professional Letter: PL/CO(92)5).
11. Department of Education and Science. *HIV and AIDS: a guide for the education service.* London: Department of Education and Science, 1991.
12. Department of Health. *Children and HIV: guidance for local authorities.* London: Department of Health, 1992.

(b) Other sexually transmitted diseases

The total number of new cases seen at GUM clinics in England in 1991 increased by just under 10% to 634,438 (see Table 6.5): sexually transmitted disease was diagnosed in just over 58%. Chlamydial and non-specific genital infection (NSGI) accounted for about 17% of cases, infection with wart virus or herpes simplex virus for about 16% and gonorrhoea for just under 3% of cases (see Figure 6.5).

There was a further fall in most non-viral sexually transmitted diseases, although there are signs that a plateau may have been reached for infections that fell most sharply in the mid 1980s. Reports of gonorrhoea, for example, fell by almost 60% between 1985 and 1988 but by less than 3% between 1988 and 1991. Recently, there was concern about increased gonorrhoea among men, but the 1991 figures indicate that there is no established upward trend (see Figure 6.6). Since the introduction in 1988 of the KC60 reporting form for consultations in GUM clinics there have been some inconsistences in reporting practice, and a review has led to revision of the gonorrhoea figures for 1988-90 (see Table 6.6). The total number of reports of gonorrhoea in 1991 fell by 7.4% to 18,683 cases; in men there was a decrease of 7.9% to 11,399, and in women a decrease of 6.6% to 7,284.

Although the total number of reports of uncomplicated chlamydial infection increased slightly, from 36,483 to 36,672, the total number of uncomplicated non-gonococcal genital infections fell due to a decrease in reports of non-specific genital infections from 75,775 in 1990 to 71,575 in 1991; this decrease was almost entirely accounted for by a 7.3% fall in the number of cases among men.

There was further increase in reports of pelvic inflammatory disease, from 5,426 in 1990 to 5,528 in 1991. As in previous years, no organism was found in most cases (84%).

There was a slight increase in reports of syphilis, largely because of a rise in non-infectious syphilis in men. Only 348 cases of infectious syphilis were reported, representing just over 25% of the total.

160

Table 6.5: *Sexually transmitted diseases reported by NHS genito-urinary medicine clinics in England in the year ended 31 December 1991*

Condition	Males	Females
All syphilis	885	464
Infectious syphilis	*238*	*110*
All gonorrhoea	11399	7284
Post-pubertal uncomplicated	*10484*	*5984*
Chancroid/Donovanosis/LGV	53	16
Other chlamydia (excluding PID and chlamydial infections with arthritis)[1]	16953	20014
Post-pubertal uncomplicated	*13694*	*16630*
Pelvic infection and epididymitis	1573	5528
Non-specific urethritis (NSU) and related disease	53348	18227
Chlamydial infections/NSU with arthritis	327	57
Trichomoniasis	334	5929
Vaginosis/vaginitis/balanitis	9933	32823
Candidiasis	9541	50094
Scabies/pediculosis	4990	1925
Herpes-all	10823	11016
Herpes simplex-first attack	*6152*	*7122*
Herpes simplex-recurrence	*4671*	*3894*
Wart virus infections-all	48225	34393
Wart virus infection-first attack	*28235*	*24439*
Wart virus infection-recurrence	*19990*	*9954*
Viral hepatitis	647	79
HIV/AIDS (first presentations)	5511	481
Asymptomatic HIV infection - subsequent presentation[2]	*7880*	*694*
Other conditions requiring treatment[3]	51904	43530
Other episodes not requiring treatment	90496	74266
Other conditions referred elsewhere	5307	6063
Total new cases seen	322249	312189

[1] Comprises "uncomplicated chlamydial infection", "other complicated chlamydia (excluding PID and epididymitis)" and "chlamydia ophthalmia neonatorum".

[2] In previous reports this category was included in the HIV/AIDS total. It has now been removed from the list of new cases and is included here for the sake of continuity.

[3] Includes epidemiological treatment of trichomoniasis, vaginosis, vaginitis, balanitis and candidiasis.

LGV = lymphogranuloma venereum; PID = pelvic inflammatory disease.

Source: Form KC60

Figure 6.5: *Cases seen at NHS genito-urinary medicine clinics, England, 1991 - breakdown by condition*

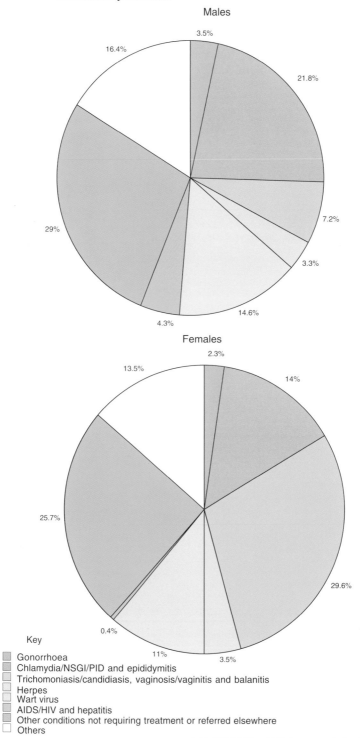

Males

3.5%
16.4%
21.8%
7.2%
3.3%
29%
4.3%
14.6%

Females

2.3%
13.5%
14%
25.7%
29.6%
0.4%
11%
3.5%

Key
- Gonorrhoea
- Chlamydia/NSGI/PID and epididymitis
- Trichomoniasis/candidiasis, vaginosis/vaginitis and balanitis
- Herpes
- Wart virus
- AIDS/HIV and hepatitis
- Other conditions not requiring treatment or referred elsewhere
- Others

Source: Form KC60

Table 6.6: *Revised figures for cases of gonorrhoea reported by NHS genito-urinary medicine clinics in England, 1988-91*

Year	Men	Women	All
1988	11080	8104	19184
1989	10994	7918	18912
1990	12380	7796	20176
1991	11399	7284	18683

Source: Form KC60

Figure 6.6: *All gonorrhoea: number of new cases seen at NHS genito-urinary medicine clinics, England, 1980-91*

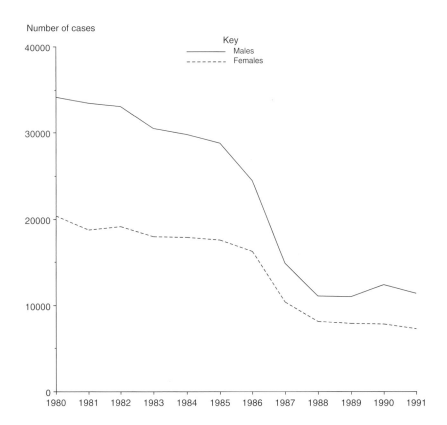

Source: Forms SBH60 and KC60

163

Wart virus and herpes simplex virus infections continued to increase, by 7.1% to 82,618 and by 8.3% to 21,839, respectively. There was a more pronounced increase in wart virus infections among men, whereas the increase in herpes simplex was greater in women. For the first time, reports of herpes simplex in women (11,016) outnumbered those in men (10,823); in 1980, less than 40% of herpes infections were found in women. For both viruses the increases in recurrent infections was greater than the increases in new infections: new cases of wart virus infection increased by 6.4% to 52,674, whilst there was an increase of 5.8% in new cases of herpes simplex to 13,274.

The growing workload related to patients with HIV infection and AIDS is reflected in a 35% increase in the number of such cases seen in GUM clinics. However, Form KC60 reports refer to consultation episodes and do not provide definitive numerical data on reported cases of HIV and AIDS. Such data are furnished by voluntary confidential reporting to CDSC (see page 150).

(c) Immunisation

Coverage

Immunisation coverage has continued to rise. By November 1992, uptake among children aged 18 months for diphtheria, tetanus and polio vaccines was 95%, and for pertussis vaccine was 91%, and uptake of measles, mumps and rubella (MMR) vaccine by the age of 2 years was 93%. New national uptake targets of 95% by 1995 were announced as part of the strategy for health[1]; of the 14 health Regions, East Anglia has already reached these targets for all vaccines and Oxford, Wessex and South Western have reached them for all vaccines except pertussis. The earlier 90% vaccination targets were reached by 95% of English health Districts for diphtheria, tetanus and polio vaccines, by 84% for MMR vaccine and by 81% for pertussis vaccine. These improved rates of achievement of targets are shown in Figure 6.7. Notifications of the matching diseases remain at historic low levels: no child in England or Wales has died of acute measles for three years and there has been only one death from pertussis since 1990. In 1992, the PHLS identified only two cases of laboratory-confirmed rubella infection in pregnant women - strong evidence that the introduction of MMR in 1988 has helped to prevent rubella infection in susceptible women during pregnancy.

Mumps-vaccine-associated meningitis

Surveillance of viral meningitis associated with the mumps vaccine component of MMR had previously indicated that one virus-positive confirmed case would occur per 225,000 distributed doses, and probable and definite cases at a rate of one per 100,000 distributed doses. This complication appeared to be associated with the Urabe strain of mumps virus present in two brands of vaccine ('Pluserix', SmithKline Beecham and 'Immravax', Merieux UK). However, studies by the PHLS[2] showed that overall meningitis rates (definite and probable cases) might be as high as one per 5,000 immunised children when laboratory data on cerebrospinal fluid samples taken from children aged 1-2 years were linked with immunisation histories held on health authority computer records. On the basis of this evidence, MMR vaccines derived from Urabe virus were no longer supplied to the NHS through central purchasing arrangements; only vaccine based on the Jeryl Lynn virus strain ('MMR-II', Merck Sharp & Dohme) is now available[3]. Many other countries that used Urabe-virus-based MMR vaccines took similar action. Research by the HEA indicates no significant change in public attitudes towards the safety of MMR vaccine, despite this announcement of a change of brands on the grounds of vaccine-associated meningitis.

Figure 6.7: *Percentages of English District Health Authorities reaching 90% immunisation targets, 1987/88 to November 1992*

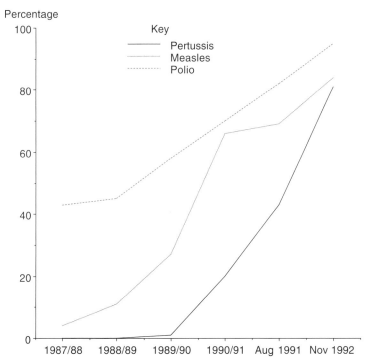

Source: DH statistics and COVER data

Haemophilus influenzae type b

In October 1992, immunisation against *Haemophilus influenzae* type b (Hib) was introduced. This vaccine is given at the same time as diphtheria, tetanus and pertussis vaccine at the age of two, three and four months. Over the first year of the programme, it is intended that all children under one year-of-age, who are most at risk of invasive Hib infection, will receive three doses; children aged between one year and four years will receive a single dose. Over 7 million doses of vaccine were needed for the first year of the programme, more than could be supplied by a single manufacturer: the total UK order comprised 5.5 million doses of Hib vaccine conjugated to tetanus toxoid (Merieux UK), and over 1.5

million doses conjugated to a diphtheria toxoid (Lederle). Because it was unknown whether the vaccines were fully interchangeable within a course of three doses, it was recommended that the Merieux vaccine could be given to any child under four years according to the above regimen, but that the Lederle vaccine should be reserved for children over one year of age who only required a single dose.

Before introduction of this vaccine, the cumulative risks for invasive Hib infection were one per 600 children under the age of five years[4]. Preliminary results from a study in the Oxford Region indicate a very high protective efficacy[5]. The national introduction of these novel vaccines was supported by a publicity campaign that included television as well as magazine and newspaper advertisements. HEA evaluation of the impact of its campaign shows an encouragingly high level of public awareness of this new childhood immunisation programme.

References

1. Department of Health. *The Health of the Nation: a strategy for health in England.* London: HMSO, 1992 (Cm. 1986).
2. Colvin A, Pugh S. Mumps meningitis and measles, mumps, and rubella vaccine. *Lancet* 1992; **340:** 786.
3. Department of Health. *Changes in Supply of Vaccine.* London: Department of Health, 1992 (Professional Letter: PL/CMO(92)11).
4. Tudor-Williams G, Frankland J, Isaacs D, et al. *Haemophilus influenzae* type b disease in the Oxford Region. *Arch Dis Child* 1989; **64:** 517-9.
5. Booy R, Moxon ER, MacFarlane JA, Mayon-White RT, Slack MPE. Efficacy of *Haemophilus influenzae* type b conjugate vaccine in Oxford region. *Lancet* 1992; **340:** 847.

(d) Hepatitis C in blood donations

During the year, 2,912,503 blood donations were screened for anti-HCV (antibody to hepatitis C virus): 12,108 (0.4%) were positive on the initial test, of which 7,745 (0.27% overall) were repeatedly positive. Supplementary testing of the repeatedly positive samples by recombinant immunoblot assay (RIBA) confirmed 970 donations (0.03% overall) to be positive; 2,379 (0.08%) gave an indeterminate result, 4,168 (0.14%) were negative, and 228 results are still awaited. The male:female ratio was 2.04:1 for donations confirmed to be HCV-positive, compared with 1.12:1 and 1.26:1 for indeterminate and negative samples, respectively.

Among new donors, 0.56% of samples were initially screen-positive, with 0.38% repeatedly positive. Unfortunately, 17% of these repeatedly positive samples from new donors have not yet undergone RIBA, but of those tested 0.12% are RIBA positive - a significantly higher proportion than is found across all donations.

It is hoped that continued improvement of screening and supplementary tests will lead to fewer false-positive results on initial screening and a much reduced number of indeterminate results.

(e) Legionellosis

In 1992, 146 cases of Legionnaires' disease among residents of England and Wales were reported to CDSC via its voluntary laboratory reporting system. As in most previous years, nearly half of these were probably acquired abroad (see Table 6.7). There were 25 deaths. Although this total represents a small increase from the unprecedentedly low final figure of 112 cases reported in 1991, it is encouraging that the number of cases associated with outbreaks remains low.

Table 6.7: *Reports of Legionnaires' disease, England and Wales, 1980-92*

Year	Total confirmed cases	Associated with travel abroad
1980	182	79
1981	142	63
1982	138	57
1983	159	48
1984	150	56
1985	210	56
1986	189	89
1987	209	109
1988	278	82
1989	240	91
1990	188	91
1991	112	52
1992	146	64

Source: The National Surveillance Scheme for Legionnaires' Disease (supplied by CDSC)

In November 1992, the Health and Safety Executive (HSE) introduced Regulations[1] requiring wet cooling towers to be registered with local authorities. It is hoped that this move will improve the standard of maintenance of cooling towers and facilitate the investigation of outbreaks. The report of the joint DH/HSE Working Group on the Prevention and Control of Legionellosis, which had been presented to the four UK Chief Medical Officers and to the Health and Safety Commission in September 1991, was subsequently published by DH[2].

References

1. Department for Employment. *The Notification of Cooling Towers and Evaporative Condensers Regulations 1992*. London: HMSO, 1992 (Statutory Instrument 1992: no. 2225).
2. Joint Health and Safety Executive and Department of Health Working Group on Legionellosis. *The Prevention and Control of Legionellosis: review and forward look. First Report to the Health and Safety Commission and Chief Medical Officers*. Heywood (Lancashire): Department of Health, 1992.

(f) Influenza

Influenza activity was low throughout 1992. During the early part of the year several different influenza viruses were circulating, but most influenza-like illness was probably caused by respiratory syncytial virus, other respiratory viruses and *Mycoplasma pneumoniae*. The absence of any major new virus strain led to the unusual decision by WHO to recommend the same vaccine strains for 1992/93 as had been used in 1991/92. For the first time, EC countries

167

met to harmonise the vaccines used within the EC and it was agreed that these WHO recommendations were appropriate for Europe. By the end of the year there was still very little influenza activity in England, but outbreaks of influenza A (H_3N_2) and some influenza B infections were being reported from China and Japan; influenza B predominated in the United States of America (USA).

Despite these low levels of activity during 1992, some influenza circulates every year and its spread is poorly understood; epidemics are therefore difficult to predict. It is important that all those in the 'at risk' groups listed in the Chief Medical Officer's annual letter on influenza immunisation[1] and in DH's memorandum, *Immunisation against Infectious Disease*[2], are protected by annual immunisation against influenza.

References

1. Department of Health. *Influenza immunisation*. Heywood (Lancashire): Department of Health 1992 (Professional letter: PL/CMO(92)12).
2. Department of Health. *Memorandum "Immunisation against infectious disease"*. Heywood (Lancashire): Department of Health, 1992 (Professional Letter: PL/CMO(92)7).

(g) Tuberculosis

During 1992, it became ever more apparent that tuberculosis is not a disease of the past. A resurgence of tuberculosis in Africa and parts of the USA has already been well documented. WHO data confirm an increase in several European countries: the main contributory factors are thought to be immigration from high incidence areas and an association with HIV infection. In England and Wales, provisional notified cases of tuberculosis increased to 5,798 in 1992, compared with 5,436 in 1991, 5,204 in 1990 and 5,432 in 1989. Although this figure is still lower than the 5,993 notifications in 1986, it is the highest recorded for six years. 334 deaths were notified in 1992 - fewer than in each of the previous two years.

Effective planning of policies and services to cope with this apparent increase in tuberculosis requires more detail about the population groups affected and trends in the incidence of the disease than is provided by the ordinary notification system. A detailed national survey of notifications of tuberculosis, referred to in last year's Report[1], will start in January 1993 under the co-ordination of CDSC. Wherever possible the survey will include anonymous HIV tests for patients with tuberculosis aged 16-54 years to assess the association between HIV infection and tuberculosis.

A cause of concern in the USA has been the number of outbreaks due to multiple-drug-resistant organisms, particularly among patients with co-existing HIV infection; the associated mortality is high. Increased drug resistance of *Mycobacterium tuberculosis* isolates in the UK has not yet been identified, but surveillance for this phenomenon has been heightened.

In the light of this experience, the 1990 decision of the Joint Committee on Vaccination and Immunisation to continue the schools' BCG immunisation programme until at least the mid-1990s appears even more prudent. Control of tuberculosis also depends on the early detection and effective treatment of infected people. DH is reviewing the arrangements for screening new entrants to the UK who come from areas with a high incidence of tuberculosis, and has funded several initiatives to improve health care among the homeless - another group at increased risk of the disease.

Reference

1.   Department of Health. *On the State of the Public Health: the annual report of the Chief Medical Officer of the Department of Health for the year 1991.* London: HMSO, 1992; 103.

(h) Shigellosis

The sudden increase in the number of notifications of *Shigella sonnei* infection during the last 10 weeks of 1991 continued into the first quarter of 1992. Although the number of notifications subsequently fell steadily, the total for 1992 was 17,000 compared with nearly 10,000 for 1991. By the end of the year the number of notifications was running at about three times the level reported in late 1990.

Because of this increase, and a lack of evidence for the efficacy of various control measures, the PHLS convened a Working Group to review transmission of shigellosis and to recommend ways to prevent its spread. The Working Group concluded that transmission was most commonly by direct person-to-person, faecal-oral spread, usually after exposure to liquid infected stool; that pre-school children and those in nursery and infant schools are at highest risk of, and most likely to transmit, the infection; and that symptomless excretion during convalescence or in apparently healthy individuals poses little risk of infection if good hygiene practices are observed.

The full recommendations of the Working Group will be published in *Communicable Disease Report* during 1993. They will emphasise the importance of hand washing after using the toilet and before meals. Schools and nurseries need to have suitable toilet facilities (with toilet paper, hand basins, soap, water and disposable hand towels or other hygienic drying facilities), and a policy for regular cleaning. Hand-washing ought to be supervised in nurseries and infant schools. Children with diarrhoea should be excluded from schools or nurseries, but can return when symptom-free and with normal stools as long as good personal hygiene is maintained; bacteriological clearance is unnecessary. Information on prevention and control measures should be made widely available to parents, teachers and carers.

(i) Travel-related disease

Travellers abroad may be exposed to a wide variety of infections. Some are diseases rarely seen in this country, particularly those associated with inadequate sanitation and conditions of poor personal and food hygiene. Others may reflect changed behaviour patterns on holiday or on work-related travel.

Immunisation

Three vaccines for travellers, one against hepatitis A and two against typhoid fever, were licensed for use in Britain during 1992.

Hepatitis A is one of the commonest infections acquired abroad. Human normal immunoglobulin has been used for some time to give good protection for up to three months. The new formaldehyde-inactivated hepatitis A virus vaccine produces immunity for at least 10 years after three injections at 0, 1 and 6-12 months, and is therefore more suitable for prolonged or frequent travel to endemic areas.

The two new vaccines against typhoid fever are no more effective in protecting against infection than the old whole-cell vaccine, but may be better tolerated. One is a single-dose injectable vaccine prepared from purified capsular antigen (the V_i or virulence antigen) of *Salmonella typhi* and produces immunity lasting three years. The other, oral, vaccine consists of live attenuated *S. typhi* organisms in a capsule that must be swallowed whole at least one hour before food; some doubts have been raised about how closely recipients will comply with the dosage schedule and the requirement to keep capsules refrigerated until taken, and about whether there are sufficient organisms in the preparation.

During 1991, there were reports from Denmark and Australia of severe allergic reactions to Japanese encephalitis vaccine. This vaccine is unlicensed in Britain, but is available on a named patient basis. Preliminary findings from a retrospective study of adverse reactions to the vaccine in recent UK recipients show no excess incidence of adverse reactions, and the vaccine will continue to be available for those at risk. One brand of Japanese encephalitis vaccine has recently been licensed in the USA.

Malaria

The PHLS Malaria Reference Laboratory has reported a total of 1,629 cases of malaria imported into the UK during 1992 - a 30% fall from the final total of 2,332 reports in 1991, and the lowest recorded for 10 years. Nevertheless, over half were caused by *Plasmodium falciparum* infection and 11 people died (compared with 12 in 1991, but only four or five annually for several preceding years). These figures underline the importance of compliance with recommended prophylaxis, including anti-mosquito measures, and the need for patients and doctors alike to recognise that no prophylactic regimen is an absolute guarantee of protection.

CHAPTER 7

ENVIRONMENTAL HEALTH AND TOXICOLOGY

(a) United Nations Conference on Environment and Development

The United Nations Conference on Environment and Development (UNCED) was held in Rio de Janeiro from 3 to 14 June 1992. Senior representatives from 172 member states attended the meeting, which culminated in the 'Earth Summit' on 12 and 13 June when 102 heads of State or Government participated.

The Department of Health (DH) contributed to the preparations for this meeting, especially with regard to chemical risk assessment and management. In December 1991, a meeting of experts was held in London to consider proposals for an inter-governmental mechanism for chemical risk assessment and management (IMCRAM). The conclusions and recommendations from this meeting were considered, and endorsed, by UNCED and subsequently by the UN General Assembly.

Agreement was reached at UNCED on the Rio Declaration on Environment and Development and on an action programme for sustained development into the next century (Agenda 21). Health concerns are principally addressed in Chapters 6 and 19 of Agenda 21, although other parts of the action programme are also relevant. Chapter 6, concerned with the protection and promotion of human health, builds on the principles that underlie the World Health Organization's (WHO's) overall strategy to work towards 'Health for All by the Year 2000', and on the work of the WHO Commission on Health and Environment. Chapter 19 covers the environmentally sound management of toxic chemicals and contains six programme areas for international collaboration:

- expansion and acceleration of the international assessment of chemicals;
- harmonisation of classification and labelling of chemicals;
- information exchange on toxic chemicals and chemical risks;
- establishment of risk reduction programmes;
- strengthening of national capabilities for the management of chemicals; *and*
- prevention of illegal international traffic in toxic and dangerous products.

It recommends that the International Programme in Chemical Safety (IPCS), in expanded form, should act as a nucleus for international co-operation in the areas covered by Chapter 19 and provide the secretariat for IMCRAM. IPCS - a joint undertaking by the UN, the International Labour Organisation and WHO - already has a key role in many of the programme areas, particularly in the assessment of chemicals. IPCS Environmental Health Criteria documents and Health and Safety Guides on the effects of chemicals on human health and the environment are internationally recognised as authoritative sources of advice. DH makes substantial contributions to the funding of IPCS and to the preparation of these documents.

Most of the areas considered in chapter 19 encompass existing work programmes of international organisations, especially the Organisation for Economic Co-operation and Development (OECD) and the European Community (EC), and it is important that the programmes of these international bodies are complementary so that work is not duplicated. DH, in close collaboration with other Government Departments, especially the Department of the Environment and the Health and Safety Executive (HSE), will lead the United Kingdom (UK) input into planning for the inter-governmental forum, which is likely to be held in April 1994.

(b) Chemical and physical agents in the environment

(i) Small Area Health Statistics Unit

The background to the establishment of the Small Area Health Statistics Unit (SAHSU) at the London School of Hygiene and Tropical Medicine was described in the Report for 1991[1]. The Unit is funded by several Government Departments to investigate claims of ill-health around point sources of industrial pollution, and to develop methodology to investigate any cluster of disease that may occur within a small area. In its first major study, SAHSU found no evidence to support claims of increased cancer risk near incinerators burning waste solvents and oil[2].

As well as responding to concerns about apparent disease clusters around industrial sites, SAHSU is carrying out investigations of particular types of industrial installation. These studies, some of which will be reported on during 1993, include investigations of the incidence of leukaemia around benzene works, and the incidence of specific cancers around municipal incinerators. In addition, the Unit has nearly completed a study of the geographical incidence of angiosarcoma of the liver in the vicinity of vinyl chloride plants in Great Britain.

Advances have been made in the methodology of analysing and interpreting health statistics in small areas, including a method to compensate for socio-economic confounding based on the Carstairs' index[3]. This is an important development because incidence rates for many diseases, including most common cancers, are related to socio-economic status; those living close to industrial installations may not be typical of the population as a whole in this respect. Other developments include the ability to analyse for multiple point sources and overlapping circles where several sources are co-located, and to incorporate routine adjustment for temporal and regional variations in completeness of postcode data and cancer registration. A detailed description of SAHSU methodology has recently been published[4].

(ii) Air pollution

DH's Advisory Group on the Medical Aspects of Air Pollution Episodes published its report on sulphur dioxide, acid aerosols and particulates in October 1992[5]. The report contained a detailed toxicological review and recommendations on the provision of advice about these pollutants to the public; a number of research recommendations were also made. The Group concluded that individuals who did not have respiratory disease would not be affected by episodes of raised sulphur dioxide concentrations such as occur in the UK. People with asthma, however, are more sensitive to sulphur dioxide and, in parts of the UK, sulphur dioxide concentrations regularly exceed those shown to induce tightness of the chest, coughing and wheezing in such individuals; these effects are acute and reversible. The Group recommended that advice be made available to the public and that a warning should be issued when concentrations of sulphur dioxide exceeded or were expected to exceed 400 parts per billion (ppb). As a result, the banding system used to describe air quality with respect to sulphur dioxide has been modified, and advice based on recommendations of the Advisory Group has been made available on a free telephone helpline (0800 556677) and on CEEFAX.

The Advisory Group reported that no firm conclusions about the effects of particulates or levels of acid aerosols could be drawn because of insufficient data. A recommendation for enhanced monitoring has been passed to the Department of the Environment.

The Advisory Group has now begun a study of the oxides of nitrogen. In December 1992, nitrogen dioxide concentrations in Manchester rose above 300 ppb - although even higher levels had been reported in London in December 1991. Such episodes are heavily dependent on meteorological conditions, and are infrequent but likely to recur. The Committee on the Medical Effects of Air Pollutants has also addressed a range of questions, including the effects of air pollutants upon asthmatics and the health effects of carbon monoxide.

The Department of the Environment's Expert Panel on Air Quality Standards has been established; these standards will be based upon a comprehensive review of the health effects of the compounds considered, and the work of DH's Advisory Group has provided a valuable starting point. Recommendations for air quality standards for ozone and benzene will be made in 1993, and recommendations for 1, 3-butadiene, sulphur dioxide, particles and nitrogen dioxide will follow.

(iii) Effects of ultraviolet radiation

In July 1992, the Committee on Medical Aspects of Radiation in the Environment (COMARE) issued a statement of advice to the Health Departments regarding the health effects of ultraviolet (UV) radiation[6]. The Committee noted with concern the recent rise in the incidence of malignant melanoma in England from 1,827 cases in 1980 to 2,635 in 1986. The much more common, though seldom fatal, non-melanotic skin cancers also increased - from 19,000 cases in 1980 to over 25,000 in 1986. The Committee considered that there was sufficient evidence to show that this rising incidence was related to exposure to UV radiation; that the risk of skin cancer was largely determined by patterns of exposure to solar UV radiation, which may be influenced by people's occupation and behaviour; and that risk varies between people of different skin type.

COMARE recommended that cancer registration procedures should be improved, and pointed to a need to inform the public of the risks of excessive exposure to sunlight. Particular attention was drawn to the need for individuals to be aware of their own skin sensitivity, to the dangers of sunburn in children and babies, and to a requirement for specific advice to be given to users of sunbeds. The Committee also noted the work of the National Radiological Protection Board Advisory Group on non-ionising radiation in identifying research needs in this area, which the Committee felt were considerable.

Skin cancer has been chosen as one of four main areas for preventive activity in the cancer key area of the strategy for health[7] (see page 68). Discussions have already taken place with the Health Education Authority (HEA) on a new national campaign, with the HSE on revised advice for users of sunbeds and with the cosmetics industry regarding the labelling of sunscreen products. A handbook for the cancer key area in the strategy for health has been prepared to help local managers institute skin cancer prevention programmes, and will be published early in 1993.

References

1. Department of Health. *On the State of Public Health: the annual report of the Chief Medical Officer of the Department of Health for the year 1991.* London: HMSO, 1992; 152.
2. Elliott P, Hills M, Beresford J, et al. Incidence of cancer of the larynx and lung near incinerators of waste solvents and oils in Great Britain. *Lancet* 1992; **339:** 854-8.
3. Carstairs V. Deprivation and health in Scotland. *Health Bull* 1990; **46:** 162-75.
4. Elliott P, Westlake AJ, Hills M et al. The Small Area Health Statistics Unit: a national facility for investigating health around point sources of environmental pollution in the United Kingdom. *J Epidemiol Community Health* 1992; **46:** 345-9.
5. Department of Health. *Sulphur Dioxide, Acid Aerosols and Particulates: report of the advisory group on the medical aspects of air pollution episodes.* London: HMSO, 1992. Chair: Professor Stephen Holgate.
6. House of Commons. Parliamentary Debate. Ultraviolet Radiation: Committee on Medical Aspects of Radiation in the Environment (COMARE). *Hansard* 1 July 1992, col 637-9.
7. Department of Health. *The Health of the Nation: a strategy for health in England.* London: HMSO, 1992 (Cm. 1986).

(c) Foodborne and waterborne diseases

Foodborne diseases

In 1992, the number of notifications of food poisoning increased by about 19%, having remained stable in the previous three years. Increases in salmonellosis and campylobacter enteritis also occurred, and the incidence of infection with verocytotoxin-producing *Escherichia coli* (VTEC) continued to rise; the reason for these increases is not known.

Advisory Committee on the Microbiological Safety of Food

The Advisory Committee on the Microbiological Safety of Food gave advice in 1992 on a definition of food poisoning for use throughout the UK. This was circulated by the Chief Medical Officer to all doctors in a letter issued in September[1]. The Committee also made good progress on its first three major studies - of *Salmonella* in eggs, vacuum packaging and associated processes, and *Campylobacter*. Reports on the first two of these were presented to Ministers towards the end of the year. Additionally, the Committee considered the strategy for its activities and decided that its future work programme should include reviews of the poultry industry, *Escherichia coli* serotype 0157, foodborne viruses and some aspects of catering. Working Groups to consider the first two of these topics were set up towards the end of the year.

Steering Group on the Microbiological Safety of Food

During 1992, the Steering Group finalised its strategy for the microbiological surveillance of food and described the ways in which this would be implemented in the short, medium and long term. Pilot and preliminary studies on microbiological contamination have already taken place or are under way for a number of foods or food areas - such as prepared salads from self-service salad bars, cream cakes, ready-to-eat meats, catering kitchen surfaces and equipment, and carcase contamination at abattoirs. A pilot study on human infectious intestinal disease has been completed and a large-scale study in England was commissioned at the end of 1992. This study should be completed in 1996.

Notifications of food poisoning

The number of cases of food poisoning (formally notified and ascertained by other means) in England and Wales reported to the Office of Population Censuses and Surveys (OPCS) in 1992 provisionally totalled 64,336 for the first 52 weeks of the year (there were 53 reporting weeks in 1992). This is an increase of 19% over the 53,881 cases provisionally reported for the same period in 1991 (the corrected figure for 1991 was 52,543; see Table 7.1). There is no obvious explanation for this increase, but the study of human infectious intestinal diseases in England will provide further information on the epidemiology of foodborne disease.

Salmonellosis

During the year, the total number of cases of human salmonellosis in England and Wales in the new Public Health Laboratory Service (PHLS) Salmonella Data Set was 31,355 (see Table 7.2). This figure is not directly comparable with the 1991 figure of 27,693 because a new reporting system for human salmonellosis came into operation on 1 January 1992. However, a comparison of the PHLS Division of Enteric Pathogens (DEP) figure for 1991 with the figure that the new system would have shown, had it been in operation then, shows a difference of less than 2%.

Table 7.1: *Food poisoning: reports to OPCS, England and Wales, 1982-92*

Year	Total*
1982	14253
1983	17735
1984	20702
1985	19242
1986	23948
1987	29331
1988	39713
1989	52557
1990	52145
1991	52543
1992	64882†

* Statutorily notified to OPCS and ascertained by other means.
† Provisional data for 53 weeks (64,336 [provisional data] for first 52 weeks).

Source: OPCS

Table 7.2: *Salmonella in human beings, England and Wales, January to December (inclusive) 1991 and 1992*

Serotype	1991		1992	
	Confirmed isolates	Acquired abroad (%)	Confirmed isolates	Acquired abroad (%)
S. enteritidis				
Phage type 4	14693	1078 *(7)*	16987	1388 *(8)*
Other phage types	2767	586 *(21)*	3107	567 *(18)*
S. typhimurium	5331	373 *(7)*	5401	456 *(8)*
Other serotypes*	4902	1511 *(31)*	5302	1392 *(26)*
S. species†	N/A	N/A	558	101 *(18)*
All serotypes	27693	3548 *(13)*	31355	3904 *(12)*

* Salmonellas fully identified as serotypes other than *S. enteritidis* or *S. typhimurium*.
† Organisms reported without further identification.
N/A Not available.

Source: PHLS Salmonella Data Set

Salmonella enteritidis remains the commonest serotype, accounting for 20,094 infections in 1992 compared with 17,460 in 1991. *Salmonella enteritidis* phage type 4 remains the commonest phage type and reports of it similarly increased from 14,693 to 16,987. Less change was seen in the number of reports of *Salmonella typhimurium* or other serotypes.

Campylobacter enteritis

The total number of laboratory reports of faecal isolations of *Campylobacter* in England and Wales made to the Communicable Disease Surveillance Centre (CDSC) in 1992 was 38,556, compared with 32,636 in 1991. This organism generally gives rise to sporadic infection: however, during 1992 two outbreaks of campylobacter enteritis involving over 200 people occurred as a result of their drinking unpasteurised milk. *Campylobacter* continues to be the commonest reported cause of bacterial gastro-enteritis in human beings.

Listeriosis

Reported cases of listeriosis in England and Wales continue at a low level. In 1992 there were provisionally 112 reported cases, compared with 126 in 1991 (see Figure 7.1).

Figure 7.1: *Reported cases of listeriosis, England and Wales, 1980-92*

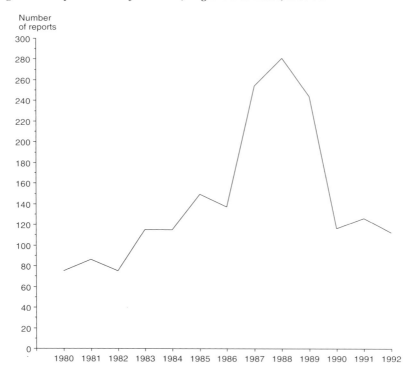

Note: 1992 data provisional.

Source: CDSC and the Division of Microbiological Reagents and Quality Control (DMRQC)

VTEC were first described in Canada in 1977[2] and were linked to an outbreak of haemorrhagic colitis in the United States of America (USA) in 1982[3]; the organisms can also give rise to the haemolytic-uraemic syndrome. In England, the first recognised outbreak of haemolytic-uraemic syndrome associated with VTEC occurred in 1984[4], and outbreaks of haemorrhagic colitis were reported in 1985[5] and 1987[6].

A few outbreaks occur each year, and some deaths have been reported in association with such outbreaks. However, most cases are sporadic and occur during the late summer months. Reports of VTEC infections have been rising over the last decade. The most common *E. coli* to cause disease in man is serotype 0157. In 1983, 6 reports of isolates of VTEC 0157 were received by the Central Public Health Laboratory for England and Wales. This rose to 468 in 1992 (see Figure 7.2). The highest incidence was in Wales and North West England, although this finding may be related to enhanced surveillance. Children and elderly people are particularly susceptible: the great majority of isolates associated with haemolytic-uraemic syndrome were from children under 10 years-of-age.

Figure 7.2: *Verocytotoxin-producing E. coli 0157, England and Wales, 1982-92*

Number of reports

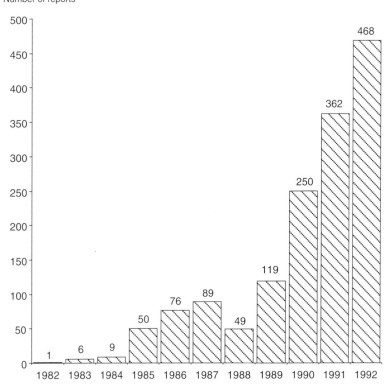

Source: PHLS LEP

VTEC 0157 has not been detected in food in the UK up to the end of 1992, but other VTEC serotypes have been identified in raw meat and sausages. Epidemiological data from some outbreaks have indicated various associations, for example with yoghurt[7] and hamburgers[8]. In one recent study, VTEC 0157 was isolated from nearly 4% of cattle arriving at an abattoir[9].

Waterborne diseases

The 1991 Annual Report of the Chief Inspector of the Drinking Water Inspectorate was published in July 1992[10]. It reaffirmed the very high quality of drinking water in this country, a finding borne out by preliminary analysis of data for 1991/92 at the PHLS CDSC. This showed that there were two confirmed waterborne outbreaks during this report period (one giardiasis, one cryptosporidiosis) and three outbreaks of cryptosporidiosis which await confirmation.

Research into the potential health effects of bathing in sewage-contaminated coastal water, jointly funded by the Departments of Health and of the Environment, the Welsh Office and the National Rivers Authority, was completed in 1992. The data accumulated from this four-year study are now being analysed and the results should be available in 1993.

References

1. Department of Health. *Definition of food poisoning.* London: Department of Health, 1992 (Professional Letter: PL/CMO(92)14).
2. Konowalchuk J, Speirs JI, Stavric S. Vero response to a cytotoxin of *Escherichia coli. Infect Immun* 1977; **18:** 775-9.
3. Riley LW, Remis RS, Helgerson SD, et al. Haemorrhagic colitis associated with a rare *Escherichia coli* serotype. *N Engl J Med* 1983; **308:** 681-5.
4. Taylor CM, White RHR, Winterborn MH, Rowe B. Haemolytic-uraemic syndrome: clinical experience of an outbreak in the West Midlands. *BMJ* 1986; **292:** 1513-6.
5. Morgan GM, Newman C, Palmer SR, et al. First recognised community outbreak of haemorrhagic colitis due to verotoxin-producing *Escherichia coli* 0157:H7 in the UK. *Epidemiol Infect* 1988; **101:** 83-91.
6. Salmon RL, Farrell ID, Hutchison JGP, et al. A christening party outbreak of haemorrhagic colitis and haemolytic uraemic syndrome associated with *Escherichia coli* 0157:H7. *Epidemiol Infect* 1989; **103:** 249-54.
7. Verotoxin producing *Escherichia coli* 0157: phage type 49. *Commun Dis Rep* 1991; **1:** 213.
8. Haemorrhagic colitis: *Escherichia coli* 0157. *Commun Dis Rep* 1991; **I:** 25.
9. Chapman PA, Siddons CA, Wright DJ, et al. Cattle as a source of verotoxigenic *Escherichia coli* 0157. *Vet Rec* 1992; **131:** 323-4.
10. Department of the Environment and Welsh Office. *Drinking Water Inspectorate. Drinking Water 1991. A report by the Chief Inspector, Drinking Water Inspectorate.* London: HMSO, 1992.

(d) Toxicological safety

(i) Dietary supplements and health foods

In 1992, following the report of the Working Group on Dietary Supplements and Health Foods[1], the Committee on the Toxicity of Chemicals in Food, Consumer Products and the Environment (COT) was asked to evaluate the safety in use of certain herbal substances.

Comfrey was the first of these substances to be assessed. Comfrey and comfrey products are available as tablets or capsules, roots, leaves and herbal teas. The

179

herb contains pyrrolizidine alkaloids - members of a large family of alkaloids, some of which are known to cause liver damage and to induce tumours in laboratory animals. There is some evidence that the alkaloids found in comfrey can cause liver damage in animals and in man.

In a recent study, the Ministry of Agriculture, Fisheries and Food (MAFF) Food Science Laboratory examined the pyrrolizidine alkaloid content of comfrey products. Generally, the highest concentrations were found in tablets (4-5 g per kg) and roots (up to 8 g per kg), whereas levels in leaf infusions and herbal teas were much lower (around 0.2-0.3% of the concentration found in tablets). COT therefore recommended that:

- the public should be warned of the potential dangers associated with the consumption of comfrey and products containing comfrey, whether commercial or home grown;

- concentrated forms of comfrey such as tablets and capsules should no longer be available;

- the public should be advised against the ingestion of comfrey root and leaves, and of teas and other infusions made from comfrey root; *and*

- comfrey teas and tinctures made from leaves may continue to be available to the public but that this recommendation should not be construed as an endorsement of such products.

COT's advice was forwarded to the Food Advisory Committee, which recommended that approaches should be made to industry to secure the voluntary withdrawal from the market of comfrey tablets and capsules (the products found to contain the highest concentrations of pyrrolizidine alkaloids) and the inclusion of a warning on product labels advising against the ingestion of comfrey root in any form (including infusions), and of comfrey leaves except in the forms of teas and infusions. Similarly, information should be made widely available to the public on the potential dangers associated with the consumption of comfrey and products in which it is used, and the matter should be drawn to the attention of the EC Commission to facilitate an EC-wide safety assessment by its Scientific Committee for Food. The EC Commission is reviewing its work programme and any EC initiative on supplements, termed dietary integrators, will depend upon the outcome.

The Government's policy continues to be that safe dietary supplements and so-called 'health' foods, even if of no nutritional value, should remain available if there is a clear public demand.

(ii) Dioxins in milk

Last year's Report[2] described how cows' milk from three farms near a local chemical works in the Bolsover area of Derbyshire was found to be contaminated with dioxins at concentrations above the Maximum Tolerable Concentration

(MTC) set by DH and MAFF. Subsequent analysis of meat from farms in the area showed that beef and offal from animals on one of these farms was also contaminated well above background levels[3]. Following advice from DH that meat from these animals should not enter the food supply, an Order under the Food and Environment Protection Act 1985 was imposed in March 1992 to prohibit movement of animals and crops from this farm. By December, however, levels of dioxins in milk and meat from all three farms had fallen significantly[4], allowing this Order to be lifted.

During 1992, people living on the three contaminated farms, and known to have consumed undiluted milk (and, in one case, eggs) asked for their blood dioxin concentrations to be measured. With the assistance of North Derbyshire Health Authority, blood samples were taken from eight individuals and analysed by MAFF scientists. The blood concentrations in these individuals ranged from 85 to 297 nanograms 2,3,7,8-tetrachlorodibenzo-p-dioxin (TCDD) Equivalency Factors per kilogram of blood fat (ng TEQs/kg fat). These levels can be compared with a mean background concentration of 41 (range 12-94) ng TEQs/kg fat in a group of people from Germany who had no known occupational exposure to dioxins[5] (there are no background data for this country). Some individuals in these families have clearly been exposed to higher than usual dioxin concentrations. However, it is thought unlikely that these concentrations will cause adverse health effects and they should fall now that exposure has been reduced to normal background levels.

(iii) Food carcinogen prioritisation

Work on the strategy for food chemical safety continued during 1992 with the development of a scheme for assigning relative priorities to potentially carcinogenic chemicals in the national food supply. For each substance dealt with by the scheme, it is envisaged that two categories of information will be required for assessment:

- an evaluation of the inherent carcinogenic hazard posed by the substance itself, as indicated by the results of toxicological testing, together with any epidemiological data; *and*

- dietary intake data to show the consumption of foodstuffs that contain the substance, and the distribution of consumers in the general population.

The Committees on the Carcinogenicity and on the Mutagenicity of Chemicals in Food, Consumer Products and the Environment (COC and COM) will advise on the carcinogenic hazards posed by substances, and MAFF has agreed to provide information about dietary intake. The separate assessments of hazard and exposure will both be taken into account when assessing the population risks associated with substances and assigning priorities.

It is anticipated that this scheme will encourage a greater concentration of regulatory activities on substances which, on objective grounds, merit most attention. The highest priorities will be accorded to those substances which possess the greatest carcinogenic potentials and to which consumers have the highest levels of exposure. In addition to man-made contaminants such as pesticide and veterinary residues, the scheme will encompass natural toxins such as patulin, aflatoxins and ochratoxin.

(iv) Advisory Committee on Novel Foods and Processes

The voluntary withdrawal from the market of germanium 'health' food supplements continued during 1992 in accordance with the advice of the Advisory Committee on Novel Foods and Processes (ACNFP), following Japanese reports of renal failure, including several deaths. At DH's request, the Medical Research Council Toxicology Unit set up a project to investigate the mechanisms that lead to germanium nephrotoxicity.

In 1992, ACNFP completed consideration of two novel foods - a specifically isolated strain of *Lactobacillus* for use as a starter culture in fermented milk products, such as yoghurt, and oils extracted from apricot and cherry kernels. The Committee advised that, provided the products met agreed specifications, they posed no food safety concerns. ACNFP also advised on a novel surveillance system that uses neutrons to scan food cargoes, and concluded that the method did not raise food safety concerns at the energies used[6].

(v) Pesticide residues in food

DH participates in the approvals process for all pesticides, and pays particular attention to the health of consumers exposed to pesticide residues in food and, in collaboration with the HSE, to the health of those involved in the manufacture or use of such compounds.

During 1992, DH and other Government Departments concerned with the control of pesticides under the Food and Environment Protection Act 1985 extended the Regulations for introducing statutory Maximum Residue Levels (MRLs) to several pesticide/crop combinations which had not been covered under earlier Regulations[7]. A revision of existing MRLs, some of which were set in 1988 on an incomplete database, is under way and will incorporate a new series of MRLs set by the EC.

The latest three-yearly report of the Working Party on Pesticide Residues[8] was published during 1992. It presented findings for the years 1988-90 and included the views of COT; the independent Committee found the results reassuring, in that residues detected would give rise to daily intakes well below acceptable levels. A notable improvement was the fall in dietary intake of organochlorine compounds, reflecting the gradual change to the use of less biopersistent insecticides on food crops. A fall in organochlorine residues in human breast milk was also reported in the Working Party's annual report for 1991[9].

(vi) Veterinary drugs

Ministers from DH and MAFF constitute the Licensing Authority for veterinary drugs. Regulations were laid before Parliament in 1991 to set legally enforceable

MRLs for such drugs. In the Regulations[10], which came into effect from 8 January 1992, MRLs were set for 24 veterinary drugs and further MRLs will be added annually.

European regulations on veterinary drugs came into force on 1 January 1992. These require that MRLs are established by the end of 1996 for all veterinary drugs currently used in food-producing animals unless it is considered that an MRL is not required to ensure human safety. No novel active ingredient may be authorised for use in food-producing animals until an EC MRL is set.

During 1992, the Veterinary Products Committee reviewed sheep dips (most of which contain organophosphates), and DH had discussions with the HSE about ways to improve work practices and the training of operatives.

(vii) Implants

DH set up a special advisory group of independent experts to review all the evidence for a possible association between the implantation of silicones (particularly silicone gel-filled breast implants) and autoimmune disease, and to advise on whether a causal relation might exist.

The group unanimously agreed that, on the basis of available data, they could find no evidence of an increased risk of connective tissue or autoimmune diseases among women who had had a silicone gel-filled breast implant, and could see no reason to alter current practice or policy. However, in view of the limited amount of data available, the group recommended that a national registry of patients with breast implants should be set up. This will be established in the Summer of 1993.

References

1. Ministry of Agriculture, Fisheries and Food and Department of Health. *Dietary supplements and health foods: report of the working group.* London: MAFF Publications, 1991.
2. Department of Health. *On the State of the Public Health: the annual report of the Chief Medical Officer of the Department of Health for the Year 1991.* London: HMSO, 1992; 159.
3. Ministry of Agriculture, Fisheries and Food. *Report of Studies on Dioxins in Derbyshire carried out by the Ministry of Agriculture, Fisheries and Food.* London: MAFF Food Safety Directorate, 1992.
4. Ministry of Agriculture, Fisheries and Food. *Third Report of Studies on Dioxins in Derbyshire carried out by the Ministry of Agriculture, Fisheries and Food.* London: MAFF Food Safety Directorate, 1992.
5. Papke O, Ball M, Lis A. Various PCDD/PCDF patterns in human blood resulting from different occupational exposures. *Chemosphere* 1992; **25:** 1101-8.
6. Advisory Committee on Novel Foods and Processes. *Report on the food safety implications of surveillance systems employing neutrons.* London: Department of Health, 1992.
7. Ministry of Agriculture, Fisheries and Food. *The Pesticides (maximum residues in food) Regulations 1988.* London: HMSO, 1988 (Statutory Instrument 1988: no. 1378).
8. Ministry of Agriculture, Fisheries and Food. *Report of the Working Party on Pesticide Residues 1988-1990.* London: HMSO, 1992 (Food Surveillance Paper no. 34).
9. Ministry of Agriculture, Fisheries and Food. *Annual Report of the Working Party on Pesticide Residues 1991: supplement to the Pesticides Register 1992.* London: HMSO, 1992. Chair: Peter Stanley.
10. Ministry of Agriculture, Fisheries and Food, Department of Health, Scottish Home and Health Department, Welsh Office. *Animals, Meat and Meat Products (Examination for Residues and Maximum Residue Limits) Regulations 1991.* London: HMSO, 1991 (Statutory Instrument 1991: no. 2843).

CHAPTER 8

OTHER EVENTS OF INTEREST IN 1992

(a) Medicines Control Agency

(i) *Role and performance*

The Medicines Control Agency (MCA) is an executive agency that reports through its Chief Executive, Dr Keith Jones, to the Secretary of State for Health. Its role is to advise Ministers and to protect the public health through the control of human medicines. Its primary concern is to ensure that medicines available to the public in the United Kingdom (UK) meet the most stringent criteria for safety, efficacy and quality. The Agency is financed by fees charged to the pharmaceutical industry but aims to set fees no higher than necessary and continuously to improve the quality of its service. It continued to be financially self-sufficient during the year, and reduced the average time for assessing licence applications for new drugs to 68 days by December 1992.

On behalf of Health Ministers (the Licensing Authority), the MCA approves medicines through the provision of a licence, monitors their use after licensing, and carries out inspection and enforcement with regard to manufacture and distribution under the provisions of the Medicines Act 1968[1], associated UK legislation and relevant European Community (EC) Directives. The MCA also supports the work of the British Pharmacopoeia Commission in setting quality standards for drug substances. The MCA has responsibility for medicines control policy within the Department of Health (DH) and represents UK interests in respect of regulatory matters within the EC and in other international settings.

During 1992, the MCA met all public health targets and eliminated a backlog of licensing applications so that important new medicines could be made available more expeditiously. Adverse Drug Reactions On-line Information Tracking (ADROIT), discussed in last year's Report[2], continued to be developed as an important new tool to assist the monitoring of adverse drug reactions in the UK. The MCA also implemented seven EC Directives and made an increased contribution to European medicines control. A five-year information technology programme was developed and legislation on good manufacturing practice was introduced.

(ii) *Control of UK clinical trials*

The UK has had legislation[1,3,4,5] to protect subjects in clinical trials since the introduction of the Medicines Act 1968[1]. Sponsors must apply to the MCA for a Clinical Trials Certificate or a Clinical Trials Exemption before a new product can be tested in patients. They must submit data from pharmaceutical and toxicological studies for assessment: if this evidence shows that the drug would not harm the trial subject, an approval is usually granted within 35 days. In 1992, applications for trials of new drugs increased by 20% to 144, of which 20% involved products of biotechnology or molecular genetics. The MCA considered 2,430 requests to extend or to vary previously approved trials, and evaluated 2,180 reports of adverse events from drugs under trial.

A new EC Directive introduced in 1992 requires all clinical trials to be conducted to good clinical practice standards if they are to be part of a Product Licence application; this move should further ensure the reliability of clinical trials data. To handle the increased workload the MCA set up a project to enhance an already extensive computer database of current clinical trials. The detailed record of the development of a drug and of its adverse drug reaction profile that can now be kept on this system has helped to place the UK at the forefront of the regulatory control of clinical trials.

(iii) Reclassification of medicines from Prescription Only to Pharmacy status

An MCA Working Party, which included representatives from the pharmaceutical profession and industry, examined procedures for reclassification of medicines so that the statutory process for removal of medicines from prescription control could be made quicker and more open. Revised guidance for applicants was published in September 1992[6]. From January 1993, there will be an annual timetable for amendments to the Prescription Only Medicines Order (the POM Order)[7]. The new guidance and timetable were explained at a seminar held jointly with the Royal Pharmaceutical Society and the Proprietary Association of Great Britain and have been well received. The Joint Working Party will meet again in 1993 to look at the scope for further improvements.

These procedural changes do not affect the requirement under the Medicines Act[1] for Ministers to consult representative interests before amendments are made to the POM Order. Those consulted include consumer and industry groups as well as a wide range of professional bodies, including the medical Royal Colleges. Ministers also have to take account of the advice of the Medicines Act advisory committees, and medicines will only be moved from POM to Pharmacy (P) status if the change can be made safely. During 1992, several medicines were moved from prescription control, including some imidazoles used locally for the treatment of vaginal candidiasis.

(iv) Developments in the European Community

The MCA has played an active part in initiatives to bring about a single European market in pharmaceuticals. In particular, the MCA negotiated and implemented a number of EC measures concerned with the licensing and control of medicines for human use.

EC licensing systems

The UK continued to take a lead in the multi-State and concertation licensing procedures (non-binding procedures to encourage and to facilitate consistent licensing decisions by EC Member States), the MCA acting as rapporteur for about a third of such procedures during the year. The MCA also had an influential role in the production of technical guidelines for pharmaceuticals in the EC.

In December, under the UK Presidency, the Internal Market Council reached agreement on future systems for medicines licensing in the EC. Two new EC licensing systems (a 'centralised' procedure for a few important high-technology medicines and a 'decentralised' procedure for other medicines, based on mutual recognition of national licensing decisions with binding arbitration in the event of disagreement) will be supported by a European Medicines Evaluation Agency. Community licensing decisions (and arbitrations) on human medicines will be based on opinions delivered by the Committee for Proprietary Medicinal Products.

The UK has long supported the principles that underlie these proposals and it has negotiated to ensure that the new procedures will embody the highest standards of public health and scientific credibility. In particular, it has pursued amendments which allow much of the responsibility for scientific assessment of products and for pharmacovigilance and inspections to remain with national authorities. The proposed European Medicines Evaluation Agency will provide technical and administrative support only. The proposals are likely to be adopted during 1993, after further consideration by the European Parliament. Implementation will then be phased in over several years.

Homoeopathic products Directive

In September, a Directive on homoeopathic medicines was adopted. It gives Member States the option to introduce a simplified registration system for certain homoeopathic products, and specific national rules can be applied to assess the safety and efficacy of homoeopathic products that do not qualify for the full registration scheme. Work is under way to implement the Directive by the end of 1993.

Implementation of other EC pharmaceutical Directives

The MCA completed implementation of the 'Extension' Directives, which bring immunological products, radiopharmaceuticals and blood products within the scope of EC medicines legislation. A Directive to introduce common standards of good manufacturing practice and Directives on the labelling and classification of medicines were also implemented.

References

1. *The Medicines Act 1968.* London: HMSO, 1968.
2. Department of Health. *On the State of the Public Health: the Report of the Chief Medical Officer of the Department of Health for the Year 1991.* London: HMSO, 1992; 149.
3. *The Medicines (Exemption from Licences) (Special Cases and Miscellaneous Provisions) Order 1972.* London: HMSO, 1972.
4. *The Medicines (Exemption from Licences) (Clinical Trials) Order 1974.* London: HMSO, 1974.

5. *The Medicines (Exemption from Licences) (Clinical Trials) Order 1981.* London: HMSO, 1981.
6. Medicines Control Agency. *Changing the legal classification of a Prescription Only Medicine for human use.* London: MCA, 1992 (MAL 77).
7. *The Medicines (Products Other Than Veterinary Drugs) (Prescription Only) Order 1983.* London: HMSO, 1983.

(b) Medical devices

Medical devices provide the technology which assists and permits the practice of modern medicine. There is a wide range, from relatively simple devices such as sutures, syringes and needles, through active implantable devices such as pacemakers and implantable defibrillators, to the feedback control systems which maintain life in intensive care units.

The role of DH's Medical Devices Directorate (MDD), which was established in August 1990, is to ensure that, as far as possible, these devices are safe and effective and that systems are in place to deal with safety, health and related problems when they occur. The MDD therefore operates a Manufacturer Registration Scheme, which covers 600-700 companies, issues advice to the National Health Service (NHS) on the safety, efficacy and use of devices, and runs a user-reporting system for device-related adverse incidents. During 1992, the MDD also published some 150 evaluation reports on a wide range of devices on the medical equipment market.

In the future, however, EC Directives will provide statutory regulation of medical devices, requiring them to comply with Essential Requirements set out in the Directives and to bear the 'CE Mark'. The Directive on Active Implantable Medical Devices will be implemented in the UK on 1 January 1993 by the Active Implantable Medical Devices Regulations 1992[1] made under Sections 11 and 27(2)(b) of the Consumer Protection Act 1987[2]. A further Directive on all other medical devices, except in-vitro diagnostic devices, received political agreement at Ministerial level at the Internal Market Council in December 1992, during the period of UK Presidency, and will take effect from 1 January 1995. A Directive on in-vitro diagnostic medical devices is being drafted.

Medical devices are generally reliable, but when they fail they can cause serious problems which may be caused by failure of the device itself, some error of a function that the device performs, or inappropriate use of the device. During 1992, the MDD received over 2,700 reports of problems, investigated over 1,000 of these in depth, and issued 24 Hazard Circulars and 67 Safety Action Bulletins. In addition, the MDD prepared a statistical analysis of risk groups for Björk-Shiley convexo-concave heart valve failures to be distributed to all relevant doctors early in 1993, investigated the ambulance transport of patients in wheelchairs or in special support seating, and continued to provide technical advice on the special initiative to provide magnetic resonance imaging, computed tomography, linear accelerators and mammography services in the NHS. In recognition of the potential for transmission of infection by contact with medical devices, MDD issued guidance on their safe use and disposal (including decontamination before further handling) and the adoption of more stringent design and production standards.

References

1. *Active Implantable Medical Devices Regulations 1992.* London: HMSO, 1992 (Statutory Instrument: SI 1992 no. 3146).
2. *The Consumer Protection Act 1987.* London: HMSO, 1987.

(c) Bioethics

(i) *Local Research Ethics Committees*

DH Guidelines issued in August 1991[1] required each District Health Authority (DHA) to establish a Local Research Ethics Committee (LREC). The task of these committees is to advise NHS bodies on the ethical acceptability of research proposals involving human subjects. The new Guidelines are much more stringent than previous arrangements, and should help to ensure increased accountability to the public; they have been widely welcomed.

All LRECs are now required to have at least two lay members, one of whom will chair their meetings or be the Chairman or Chairwoman's deputy. Membership is drawn from a wide range of groups including hospital medical staff, nursing staff, general practitioners (GPs) and lay persons. Whenever research is proposed, an LREC will look after people's best interests by careful examination of important issues such as recruitment of participants, the scientific merits of the study, consent, confidentiality and safety to ensure that the proposed research is ethical and that participants are protected.

DH keeps these arrangements under continual review. Ways to streamline the procedures to ease the process of ethical approval for multicentre research that spans a large number of Districts are being considered.

(ii) *Bioethics in Europe*

The Council of Europe has been active in bioethics since 1976, and in 1985 set up the Ad Hoc Committee on Bioethics (CAHBI). CAHBI has produced a number of recommendations and opinions which have influenced the field of bioethics not only in Europe but also further afield: these include recommendations on prenatal genetic screening and prenatal genetic diagnosis[2], and on medical research on human beings[3].

During 1992, CAHBI became the Steering Committee on Bioethics (CDBI). CDBI, like its predecessor, is charged by the Committee of Ministers to study the impact of progress in biomedical sciences on law, ethics and human rights. A working party, chaired by Dr Michael Abrams (formerly Deputy Chief Medical Officer), is developing proposals for a framework bioethics convention to consider and make recommendations about the protection of human rights and the dignity of human beings with regard to the application of biology in medicine. Another working party, chaired by Mr Peter Thompson (Solicitor to DH), is developing a specific protocol for a proposed convention on organ transplantation.

References

1. Department of Health. *Local Research Ethics Committees.* Heywood (Lancashire): Department of Health, 1991 (Health Service Guidelines: HSG(91)5).
2. Council of Europe Committee of Ministers. *Recommendation no R(90)13 on prenatal genetic screening, prenatal genetic diagnosis and associated genetic counselling.* Council of Europe: Strasbourg, 1990.
3. Council of Europe Committee of Ministers. *Recommendation no R(90)3 concerning medical research on human beings.* Council of Europe: Strasbourg, 1990.

(d) Medical manpower and education

(i) *Junior doctors' hours*

Considerable progress was made during 1992 towards achievement of the changes outlined in the 'New Deal' on hours worked by junior hospital doctors[1]. Key features of the New Deal were new working arrangements and explicit limits on contracted hours of duty for junior doctors. It set a clear timetable for change. Maximum average weekly contracted hours for junior doctors working full or partial shifts were to be reduced to 60 and 72, respectively, as soon as practicable, and to 56 and 64, respectively, by 31 December 1994. For doctors working on-call rotas, maximum average weekly contracted hours were to be reduced to 83 as soon as practicable and, for those in hard-pressed posts, to 72 by 31 December 1994.

To support the initiative, the 1991/92 funding of 200 extra consultant posts and 50 additional staff grade posts continued, alongside new funding for a further 150 consultant and 100 staff grade posts during 1992/93. These posts are part of a rolling programme, and are being established in areas where they will best facilitate reductions in junior doctors' hours. A further incentive to adopt the new working arrangements, and thus reduce excessive hours, was provided by new pay rates for out-of-hours work, introduced on 1 February 1992, which vary from 50% to 100% of basic rates according to the practitioner's working pattern.

Local assistance and advice on implementation of the New Deal is provided by Regional Task Forces, which report regularly to the Ministerial Group on Junior Doctors' Hours. Their second reports, giving staffing levels at 28 February 1992, showed the number of junior doctors contracted for more than a maximum average of 83 hours per week had fallen to 5,275. In the light of this progress, a target date of 1 April 1993 was set for the first phase of hours reductions. Regional Task Force reports giving staffing levels at 31 August 1992 revealed further progress: of 25,274 junior hospital doctors, only 3,234 remained contracted for more than 83 hours per week - a fall of over 10,000 since the medical and dental manpower census of 30 September 1990.

(ii) *'Achieving a Balance'*

Achieving a Balance: plan for action[2], published in 1987, outlined a package of measures to improve patient care and the hospital medical staffing career structure by the establishment of a more consultant-based service. Its main measure was to maintain an expansion in the number of consultant posts by at least 2% annually over 10 years. The increase in the number of consultants in post has exceeded this target, and averaged 2.8% annually from 1986 to 1991

189

when the effect of centrally funded initiatives (such as the 100 consultant posts announced in the White Paper *Working for Patients*[3]) are taken into account. The most recent central initiative has been the funding of 200 consultant posts during 1991/92, and 150 during 1992/93, to help to reduce junior doctors' hours of work. *Achieving a Balance* envisaged that 200 staff grade posts would be established annually in England and Wales over the first five years of the programme. This rate was accelerated to help to reduce junior doctors' hours. Thus 1,195 posts have now been allocated, including 50 centrally funded posts during 1991/92 and 100 in 1992/93.

The Joint Planning Advisory Committee has completed its initial scrutiny of registrar numbers. Regional quotas for NHS full-time career registrars in all specialties were completed by March 1992 and further reviews, by specialty, will be conducted every three years. Reviews of senior registrar posts continue at three-yearly intervals; most specialties have been reviewed at least twice. Quotas for part-time posts were issued by January 1991, and quotas for academic and research posts are under review.

When *Achieving a Balance: Plan for Action* was published, Regions were required to limit the number of senior house officer posts to quotas that had been agreed in 1982/83, although it was envisaged that some increases might be needed from time to time. The most recent, and largest, increase was in November 1992 in response to the findings of the Regional Task Force reports which gave staffing levels at 28 February and 31 August 1992.

(iii) Women doctors and their careers

More than 50% of students who entered medical school in the UK in September 1992 were women. During the year there was a continued emphasis on the enhancement of career opportunities for women doctors, and women doctors have also been able to take advantage of improved opportunities for flexible training.

The percentage of women consultants in surgical specialties is much lower than in most other branches of medicine. DH continued to provide funding for the Women in Surgical Training (WIST) scheme, a joint initiative with the Royal College of Surgeons of England which aims to identify and to encourage women who enter the surgical specialties by means of mutual support groups and Regional advisers.

The promotion of equal opportunities within the NHS remains a priority, and Regions have been encouraged to hold workshops to raise awareness on this issue. DH also contributed £5,000 in 1992/93 towards the production of a video on equal opportunities in relation to medical and dental recruitment.

(iv) Flexible training

DH is keen to improve the availability of flexible training opportunities for doctors. A scheme to promote the establishment of new part-time career registrar posts has been in operation since 1991, and nearly £2 million were provided for this scheme in 1992/93.

The Joint Working Party on Flexible Training has been considering the best means to meet the need for flexible training in all hospital training grades, but especially at senior registrar and senior house officer level. The Joint Working Party's report will be published early in 1993, and will set out ways to improve arrangements for flexible training, particularly for senior registrars.

(v) New career structure for doctors in community child health

The Joint Working Party on Medical Services for Children, which included representatives of the Conference of medical Royal Colleges, the British Medical Association (BMA) and DH, reported in November[4]. The Working Party's principal recommendation was that a unified career structure in child health should be achieved by the assimilation of Senior Clinical and Clinical Medical Officer grades into the mainstream medical career structure. Such a change would help to establish a combined child health service in which all medical staff receive training and continuing education in acute and preventive aspects of paediatric medicine. The report was welcomed and the NHS Management Executive will publish guidance on its implementation.

(vi) Postgraduate and continuing medical education

At the end of the year, the Secretary of State for Health agreed the recommendations of the first formal review of the Standing Committee on Postgraduate Medical Education (SCOPME), the independent advisory body on postgraduate and continuing medical and dental education. Most respondents to the formal consultation that underpinned the review warmly praised SCOPME's performance and the quality of its advice and publications. The Committee's authority has been renewed and its membership is to be increased.

Ministers also accepted the findings of a report by the joint NHS Management Executive/NHS Working Group on the Funding of Medical and Dental Training Grade Posts, which recommended a new system for the funding of hospital training posts to operate on an interim basis from 1 April 1993[5]. The key feature of the new arrangements is that part of the cost of employing training grade doctors will be met from a Regional budget, which should help to safeguard training opportunities for junior doctors yet also reduce the impact of the uneven distribution of training costs on service contract prices. The membership of the Working Group was increased to allow greater representation of provider units and the medical Royal Colleges. The larger Working Group, which held its first meeting in December 1992, is now considering how to bring greater precision to funding arrangements and the feasibility of introducing competitive training contracts; final arrangements should, it is hoped, be in place by April 1995.

During 1992, progress was made to strengthen further the arrangements to provide postgraduate and continuing medical education as set out in *Working for Patients: Postgraduate and Continuing Medical and Dental Education*[6]. Protected budgets totalling £6.061 million were allocated to Regional Postgraduate Deans to support the development of a Regional infrastructure and for medical education initiatives.

A new system of remuneration was introduced for general practice course organisers, who arrange postgraduate education for vocational trainees. From 1 April 1992, course organisers have been paid for up to two sessions per week under contract to the Regional Health Authority (RHA); previously, they were paid a flat-rate trainers' grant. A commitment was given to the BMA to enter into further negotiation early in 1993 on an improved structure for the postgraduate education of GPs, including the introduction of formal payment arrangements for GP tutors, who are responsible for the continuing medical education of GPs.

(vii) Working Group on Specialist Medical Training

A Working Group on Specialist Medical Training was established in September 1992, under the Chairmanship of the Chief Medical Officer, to consider the arrangements for specialist medical training and accreditation in the UK in the light of the requirements of EC Directives. The Working Group carried forward its work through three subgroups: these examined the structure and content of specialist training programmes; the arrangements for appointment to a consultant post; and the means by which the UK liaises with the EC on medical training and workforce issues.

The Working Group supported the development of structured and planned training programmes, and noted the potential for the duration of specialist training to be reduced. It also considered new arrangements for the award of the UK Certificate of Completion of Specialist Training and the use of a specialist indicator on the Medical Register. Its recommendations, due to be published for wider consultation in the Spring of 1993, will aim to maintain current standards of specialist training and practice and help to ensure that the UK fully meets the requirements of EC legislation.

(viii) Undergraduate medical and dental education

During 1992, the Steering Group on Undergraduate Medical and Dental Education and Research - set up to monitor the effects of the NHS reforms on, and to assess the arrangements for, teaching and research - considered important topics including academic general practice, information requirements, and a review of the arrangements for funding via the Service Increment for Teaching and Research (SIFTR). The report on the third stage of the review of SIFTR[7] was published in September 1992. Among other findings, it concluded that work to improve the sub-Regional distribution of SIFTR should continue.

As a result of the Steering Group's work, a new initiative provided £2 million from NHS regional funds to relieve service pressures on academic general practices and thus release more time for teaching and research. During the year, university departments of general practice also received £460,000, their third payment from a fund set up in 1990.

(ix) Medical Manpower Standing Advisory Committee

Planning the Medical Workforce[8], the first report of the Medical Manpower

Standing Advisory Committee, was published in December 1992. It identified the likelihood of a shortfall of doctors over the next 10-20 years and recommended encouragement of initiatives on flexible working to increase retention of trained doctors; an increase in the annual medical school intake of 240 to 4,470 places by October 1994, including an increase in the quota of overseas students; and further research to examine the manpower effects of skill-mix initiatives, the career patterns of doctors, and the affordability of further increases in the medical workforce.

References

1. Department of Health. *Hours of Work of Doctors in Training: the new deal*. London: Department of Health, 1991 (Executive Letter: EL(91)82).
2. Newton T, Grabham AH, Roberts G. *Hospital Medical Staffing: Achieving a Balance: plan for action: a report issued by the steering group for implementation on behalf of the UK Health Departments, the Joint Consultants Committee and the Chairmen of Regional Health Authorities*. London: Department of Health and Social Security, 1987.
3. Department of Health. *Working for Patients: the NHS review*. London: HMSO, 1989 (Cm. 555).
4. NHS Management Executive/British Medical Association. *Report of the Joint Working Party on Medical Services for Children*. London: Department of Health, 1992.
5. Department of Health. *Funding of hospital medical and dental training grade posts*. London: Department of Health, 1992 (Executive Letter: EL(92)63).
6. Department of Health. *Working for Patients: postgraduate and continuing medical and dental education*. Heywood (Lancashire): Department of Health, 1991.
7. Department of Health. *Review of the Service Increment for Teaching and Research (SIFTR): report on Stage 3*. London: Department of Health, 1992 (Finance Directorate Letter: FDL(92)85).
8. Medical Manpower Standing Advisory Committee. *Planning the medical workforce*. Heywood (Lancashire): Department of Health, 1992. Chair: Professor Colin Campbell.

(e) The Tomlinson Report

Sir Bernard Tomlinson and his Inquiry Group were asked to advise on the organisation of health care and medical education and research in London. The Group's terms of reference were: "To advise the Secretaries of State for Health and Education and Science on how the relevant statutory authorities are addressing the provision of health care in inner London, working within the framework of the reformed NHS, including the balance of primary health services; and the organisation and provision of undergraduate medical teaching, postgraduate medical education and research and development; taking account of:

-   the health needs of London's resident and day time population;

-   the emerging purchasing plans of health authorities and their likely impact on inner London hospitals;

-   future developments in the provision of acute and primary care; *and*

-   the need to maintain high quality patient care and, as a foundation for this, high standards of medical teaching, research and development".

The Report was published in October 1992[1], and was welcomed by the Government, whose detailed response will be published early in 1993. The key recommendations of the Report included:

- a shift of resources from acute hospitals to primary and community health services, to bring standards of primary health care up to those found elsewhere (GP premises were identified as in particular need of improvement), and to enable rationalisation of hospital services in inner London;

- the designation of a special primary care development zone in London which would assist the development of a better service in line with local health needs;

- greater variety in methods of delivering primary and community care, and alternative models such as the location of GPs in hospital accident and emergency departments and the creation of extended local health centres;

- the restructuring of 'whole-District' Trusts to separate acute and community services;

- a reduction in the bed capacity of London hospitals to match increasing efficiency and the fall in referrals of patients from outside London;

- a rationalisation of the many dispersed specialist services, merging some teaching hospitals and Trusts and closing some hospital sites;

- the full integration of Special Health Authorities into the internal market as NHS Trusts, so that they could compete on a level playing field for service contracts and for support for research and teaching, whilst securing the necessary flows of patients with rare illnesses;

- modified funding regimens to enable funds for teaching and research to be available competitively to any hospital that supported research and postgraduate teaching;

- amalgamation of medical schools and postgraduate institutions into four multi-faculty colleges of London University to improve medical education and research; *and*

- effective management of change by the setting up of an Implementation Group to follow through the recommendations and to secure effective co-ordination of a restructured NHS in London.

As part of the Government's response to the Inquiry, a London Implementation Group will be set up to take forward these recommendations. This Group will operate through existing health agencies and work closely with purchasers and providers of health care and other key bodies including the Higher Education Funding Council for England.

Reference

1. Department of Health, Department for Education. *Report of the Inquiry into London's Health Service, Medical Education and Research: presented to the Secretaries of State for Health and Education by Sir Bernard Tomlinson.* London: HMSO, 1992.

(f) Dental health

(i) *Dental health of the nation*

Provisional results from surveys conducted by DHAs in 1991/92 indicate very
small increases in the mean numbers of decayed and missing primary teeth and a
very small fall in the mean number of filled primary teeth in 5-year-old children
since 1989/90, although individual Districts show various patterns. The
proportion of filled teeth to decayed, missing and filled teeth is commonly used
as a measure of the level of restorative dental provision: over the two years since
1989/90, this measure has fallen from 20.6% to 18.4% in this age-group, but the
data must be interpreted with great caution because of differences in examination
methods and inter-examiner variability. It would be wrong to attempt to draw
any firm conclusions from this preliminary analysis, but the small changes which
seem to have occurred are undesirable and these trends will need to be closely
monitored.

Preliminary findings from the 1991 General Household Survey confirm that the
proportion of edentulous adults continues to fall quite rapidly: 17% of all adults
aged 16 years and over in Great Britain had no natural teeth, compared with 26%
in 1983.

(ii) *General dental services*

At the end of September 1992, two years after introduction of the new dental
contract, over 7 million children under the age of 18 years and 21.8 million
adults had been registered with general dental practitioners under a capitation or
continuing care arrangement. These figures represent 65% and 59%,
respectively, of the relevant population and had increased from 5.8 million
children and 15.6 million adults in September 1991.

This increased uptake of general dental services (GDS) was achieved against the
background of a dispute between DH and the dental profession. In 1991/92,
payments to dentists were much higher than had been expected; the available
evidence indicated that, if the fee-scales in operation on 1 July 1991 were left
unchanged, dentists would receive substantially more in net income than had
been recommended by the Doctors and Dentists' Review Body. In response, the
Secretary of State for Health set up a fundamental review of the system of dental
remuneration by Sir Kenneth Bloomfield. In July 1992, a 7% reduction in fees
was announced, together with a reduction from £600 to £200 of the threshold of
treatment costs above which dentists must seek prior approval from the Dental
Practice Board. It was anticipated that this decision, which was reached in the
light of all available evidence and after consultation with the dental profession,
would still deliver a target average net income in excess of the 8.5% increase that
had been recommended.

As a result of these changes, some dentists decided not to accept certain patients,
and in some areas patients have had difficulty in obtaining NHS dental services.

The Government has been determined to take whatever steps are necessary to ensure that dental services remain available in the NHS and have reminded all Family Health Services Authorities of their power to appoint salaried dentists where necessary. By the end of 1992, 65 salaried dentists were in post in England. Sir Kenneth Bloomfield's Report identifies a range of options for change, to be considered in consultation with the profession and other interested parties[1].

(iii) Community dental services

The role of the community dental services was redefined in 1989[2] with the intention that the GDS should take prime responsibility for the maintenance of oral health care for the family. During 1992, difficulties arising from the dental dispute created extra demands on community dental services.

Following acceptance by the Health Departments of the principal clinical recommendations on general anaesthesia, sedation and resuscitation in dentistry, made by the Standing Dental Advisory Committee[3], DHAs were required during 1992 to review the provision of dental general anaesthesia to ensure that local needs were met most effectively. In particular, it was felt necessary to react to the reduced availability of treatment under general anaesthesia in general dental practice, and preliminary evidence indicates a valuable contribution to such provision by the community dental services.

The new Form KC64, introduced in 1990/91, has replaced the 28M series of returns for the collection of community dental service statistics. These data will provide valuable information on screening and preventive programmes, patient care and hours worked within the community dental services; as the database builds more information should also become available on referral rates to and from the GDS.

Sir Kenneth Bloomfield's review of dental remuneration, published in December 1992[1], takes into account the activity of the community dental services and suggests closer co-operation, or even amalgamation, with the GDS.

(iv) Hospital dental services

The number of hospital dentists in England fell by 1.5%, from 1,201 whole-time equivalent posts to 1,183, between September 1990 and September 1991. The number of consultants in post remained at 400; however, the number of senior registrars fell by 10% from 112 to 101 and the number of senior house officers by 1% from 229 to 227.

Compared with 1990/91, there was a rise in new outpatient referrals to consultant clinics in three dental specialties during 1991/92: referrals rose by 25.2% from 44,789 to 56,084 in restorative dentistry; by 48.2% from 16,686 to 24,719 in paediatric dentistry and by 6.5% from 86,834 to 91,464 in orthodontics. Numbers of referrals in oral surgery fell by 3.1% to 379,496 in 1991/92, compared with 391,566 in 1990/91.

(v) Continuing education and training for dentists

The voluntary vocational training schemes for the GDS, which commenced in 1988, continued to expand. By December 1992, there were 330 trainees in 35 regionally-based programmes; five other programmes are due to start during 1993. Vocational training will become mandatory for the GDS in October 1993.

The Committee for Continuing Education and Training identified the following topics as priority areas for GDS postgraduate training in 1992: 'hands-on' courses; the management of elderly or disabled patients and those with special needs; venepuncture; the training of trainers, examiners and advisers; and courses to reinforce central initiatives. The Regional Postgraduate Dental Deans organised these courses under Section 63 arrangements[4].

During the year, central training initiatives included the production and distribution of two videotapes - *Medico-Dental Matters*, which related to medical histories, and *The Millman Street Case Book*, which dealt with communication between dentists, practice staff and dental technicians. The Teamwork Project[5] was continued, a pilot project was set up to develop and evaluate three computer-assisted learning programmes in three Regions, and the project *Pathways in Practice* was developed in collaboration with the Faculty of General Dental Practitioners of the Royal College of Surgeons of England.

(vi) Dental research

Diet and the dental health of young children

The Office of Population Censuses and Surveys (OPCS) was commissioned to conduct a national survey of the dental health and diet of young children aged 1-4 years. Approximately 1,500 children, selected at random in England, Scotland and Wales, are being examined in four equal groups at three-monthly intervals. The survey is carried out in the child's home and consists of a simple dental examination (to note, among other data, the presence of caries, trauma to the incisors and erosion of the upper incisors) together with a dental and dietary questionnaire. Fieldwork for the dental examination is being organised by the University of Birmingham Dental School.

Data from this survey will be correlated with information gathered from a more detailed nutritional survey of the same sample group, which is running concurrently and includes a weighed four-day dietary analysis and blood analysis.

Glove wearing

The University of Manchester has published further results from a commissioned longitudinal study into the changing pattern of the use of, and the difficulties experienced with, non-sterile gloves in general dental practice[6]. Some 84% of dentists in England and Wales are now wearing gloves on a routine basis, compared with 69% in 1989; however, 26% of glove wearers reported unspecified skin irritation and 13% had noted an allergic reaction to gloves in one or more of their patients.

References

1. Department of Health. *Fundamental Review of Dental Remuneration: report of Sir Kenneth Bloomfield KCB.* London: Department of Health, 1992.
2. Department of Health. *Health Services Management. The future development of Community Dental Services.* Heywood (Lancashire): Department of Health, 1989 (Health Circular: HC(89)2).
3. Standing Dental Advisory Committee. *General anaesthesia, sedation and resuscitation in dentistry. Report of an Expert Working Party.* London: Department of Health, 1990. Chair: Professor David Poswillo.
4. *Health Services and Public Health Act 1968.* London: HMSO, 1968.
5. Seward M, ed. *Teamwork: Dental Practice Training Folder, vol 2.* London: British Dental Journal, 1992.
6. Burke FJT, Wilson NHF. Allergic reactions to rubber gloves in dental patients. *Br Dent J* 1992; **173:** 124.

CHAPTER 9

INTERNATIONAL HEALTH

(a)   Britain, Europe and health

Many of the health challenges encountered in England and the United Kingdom (UK) as a whole are also found in the rest of Europe. Diseases have little respect for national boundaries, and ageing populations, technological advances and increased expectations inexorably lead to greater demands on a nation's health services. But the fact that these challenges are faced together is a source of great hope. The cumulative experience in dealing with health issues in the European Community (EC), with a population of 340 million, is vast. If put to best use, this knowledge will benefit not only EC citizens but also those in the wider Europe and the rest of the world.

The international aspects to health care are diverse, as are the international bodies involved in this work - of which the EC, the Council of Europe, the Commonwealth and the World Health Organization (WHO) are the most important to the UK. Nowhere can be insulated from the huge changes taking place in the world. In 1992, Bulgaria became the latest Eastern European member of the Council of Europe; Georgia and Slovenia were admitted to full membership of WHO; and the EC Summit in Edinburgh approved the opening of negotiations for further enlargement of the EC. The UK has an important role in all these institutions. Whatever the future holds, common approaches to common problems will be of common benefit.

(b)   The European Community

(i)   EC Presidency health initiatives

The UK held the EC Presidency from 1 July 1992 until 1 January 1993. Its main health initiative was to set out a framework for future Community action on public health, which has until now tended to grow in a piecemeal fashion. The UK encouraged the Council of Health Ministers, when considering future European action on public health, to take greater account of factors external to health systems - such as smoking, diet or the consumption of alcohol - which are not generally amenable to medical or scientific intervention. The framework paper presented by the European Commission at the Council also addressed ways to encourage disease prevention and the promotion of good health by public education, research and exchange of information. EC Health Ministers affirmed the importance of a public health framework to ensure greater continuity and coherence to Community health policies. Denmark and Belgium, who will hold the Presidency during 1993, have agreed to continue its development.

A Resolution on the monitoring and surveillance of communicable diseases was agreed. The optimum co-ordination of Member States' systems for identification of, and responses to, outbreaks of communicable disease is an important goal, particularly in view of the increased movement of goods and people within the single market.

A Memorandum on ways to reduce smoking in the Community set out all available approaches, including health education, tobacco pricing and taxation, labelling of tobacco products and controls on tobacco advertising. The UK's aim was to ensure that the Council of Health Ministers took the widest possible view of this problem. EC partners welcomed the debate and Denmark undertook to examine further the impact of pricing policies on cigarette consumption during its Presidency.

In November, the Council of Health Ministers launched the first European Drug Prevention Week. The UK Presidency took a strong lead in the organisation of this event; it included a conference which provided a valuable forum for professionals to exchange information and practical experience in prevention activities. Many other events were held at national and local level across the Community.

(ii) Treaty on European Union (Maastricht)

The Government has welcomed the new public health article (Article 129) of the Maastricht Treaty, which provides for Community activity on disease prevention and health promotion. The Article will clarify the legal base for Community activity in this field, and will allow the development of a more coherent approach to co-operation on public health issues. EC action will be confined to encouraging co-operation between Member States and supporting their activities, and will take the form of 'incentive measures' and recommendations. Harmonisation of Member States' laws is ruled out and Member States will remain responsible for the health of their citizens and the provision of health care services. The principle of subsidiarity will apply, under which Community action takes place only if (and only to the extent) justified under guidelines which were adopted at the Edinburgh European Council.

Under the terms of the Article, the Community and Member States will also be expected to foster co-operation with other countries and relevant international organisations such as WHO. Decisions under the new Article will be taken by qualified majority voting. Health is one of the areas where 'incentive measures' would be subject to the new negative assent procedure, under which the European Parliament will have ultimate power to block measures.

The new Article refers to the need to ensure that health promotion forms part of the Community's other policies. Of course, EC measures with an impact on public health have been adopted in the past, in areas as diverse as pharmaceuticals, medical devices, food safety, research, and medical qualifications.

(iii) European Economic Area

The EC and the European Free Trade Association (EFTA) signed an Agreement on the creation of a European Economic Area (EEA) at the EC Foreign Affairs

Council on 2 May 1992. This Agreement will extend most of the EC Single Market principles to the EFTA member countries (Austria, Finland, Iceland, Liechtenstein, Norway, Sweden and Switzerland) and was due to come into effect by 1 January 1993 subject to ratification by the EC, EFTA and Member States. Implementation was delayed because Switzerland voted against participation in the Agreement in a referendum held on 6 December 1992. Negotiations are under way to revise the Agreement, which is expected to come into force during 1993.

(iv) The Council of Health Ministers

There were two meetings of the Council of Health Ministers during the year. The first was held on 15 May under the Presidency of Portugal. The main developments were in tobacco and drug abuse. The second Directive on tobacco labelling was adopted: it extends previous legislation on health warnings to tobacco products other than cigarettes, and bans the marketing of oral snuff in the Community. A Declaration carrying forward work on the European Drug Prevention Week was also agreed.

The second meeting was held under the UK Presidency. The agenda and achievements of that Council meeting on 13 November are described on page 199.

(v) EC/WHO/Council of Europe

Several EC members, including the UK, have recognised for some time that working relations between the Community and WHO could be strengthened. The WHO European Regional Committee set up a committee to look into these relations. The main conclusions of the committee's report, approved by the WHO Regional Committee meeting in Copenhagen in September, were that

- There should be a new WHO European Region standing committee to act for, and in support of, the WHO European Regional Committee in its policy and supervisory roles; *and*

- There should be gradual rapprochement between the main organisations within the European region - the WHO, the EC, and the Council of Europe.

The matter was discussed briefly at the EC Council of Health Ministers in November, when the opportunity to discuss future co-operation with the WHO European Regional Committee and the Council of Europe was welcomed.

(vi) Echo

The first issue of the Department of Health's (DH's) international newsletter, *Echo*, appeared in May 1992. Published nine times a year and produced by DH's International Relations Unit, *Echo* includes news items and more detailed articles on a broad range of international health and social services topics. The emphasis is on EC matters, but there is coverage of other international issues arising, for example, from the work of WHO and the Council of Europe. Over 18,000 copies are distributed to managers in the National Health Service (NHS), professional organisations, Members of the European Parliament, and colleagues overseas.

(vii) Free movement of people

Working Group on Specialist Medical Training

A Working Group was formed under the Chairmanship of the Chief Medical Officer to advise UK Ministers on any action needed to bring the UK into line with EC law on specialist medical training (see page 192). A report is due to be made to the Secretary of State for Health in the Spring of 1993.

Health professionals

The number of health professionals from other Member States working in the UK is small and most come for short periods to gain experience. In 1992, 1,053 doctors with qualifications from other Member States obtained full registration with the General Medical Council, 70 dentists with the General Dental Council, 22 pharmacists with the Royal Pharmaceutical Society of Great Britain and 620 nurses and 21 midwives with the UK Central Council for Nursing, Midwifery and Health Visiting.

Patients

EC Social Security Regulation 1408/71 continued to operate satisfactorily, co-ordinating health care cover for people moving between Member States. The main categories covered were temporary visitors, detached workers and pensioners transferring their residence to another Member State. In 1992, 463 applications by UK patients for referral to other Member States specifically for treatment of pre-existing conditions were approved by DH. About 370 citizens of other Member States were treated in the UK on the same basis.

(viii) Directive on data protection

During the year a draft EC Directive on Data Protection was circulated to Member States for comment. In the UK, the confidentiality of personal health information is protected by duties in common law and the ethical obligations of health professionals. Processing, including individuals' rights of access to their own personal information, is subject to the Data Protection Act 1984[1] and the Access to Health Records Act 1990[2], both of which contain specific safeguards.

The Department consulted widely on the draft EC Directive which, if adopted, would have considerable implications for the processing of personal health data. The consultation showed wide concern about the effects of the proposed

Directive, and these anxieties have been conveyed to the European Commission. There will be further discussions during 1993 about this proposed Directive.

(ix) 'Europe Against Cancer'

'Europe Against Cancer' is the EC campaign which was launched in 1985 with the aim of reducing expected cancer mortality in Member States by 15% by the year 2000. The programme's main themes are prevention, public information and education, training and co-ordination of research.

DH has supported UK projects under this programme for several years and a further £161,000 were made available for 1992/93. Each year, the programme has a specific theme. In 1992 a week of activities centred on 'Cancer Prevention and Health Promotion in the Workplace', and publicising the programme's other messages, was held in October.

(x) Smoking

The Council of Health Ministers adopted a second Directive on tobacco labelling, which extends stronger health warnings to tobacco products other than cigarettes and bans oral snuff. The proposed EC Directive to ban all tobacco advertising continued to be discussed at Council Working Groups, but without agreement.

During its Presidency, the UK introduced a Memorandum on strategies for reducing tobacco consumption. The Memorandum to the Council of Health Ministers was a systematic investigation of the different anti-smoking policies used in Member States, with a discussion of where future action could be concentrated. The European Commission also published a Report on smoking in public places, to be discussed at future Council meetings.

(xi) Elderly and disabled people

Progress was made during the UK Presidency towards reaching agreement on HELIOS II, the third EC Action Programme to assist disabled people. The Handynet disability database became available on CD-ROM (compact disc read-only memory).

The 1993 'European Year of Older People and Solidarity between Generations' was officially launched in the UK by the Secretary of State for Health at the 1992 Age Resource Awards on 17 December 1992. Plans were laid for a full programme of events and activities to celebrate the Year, which aims to raise awareness of issues of ageing, to promote positive images of older people and a closer relationship between generations, and to facilitate the exchange of good practice across Europe.

(xii) AIDS and HIV infection

In December 1992, as part of the UK's EC Presidency activities, the Health Departments hosted a symposium on the future direction of HIV and AIDS programmes in Europe. It was attended by delegates from many European countries, including those in Central and Eastern Europe, and a key-note speech was given by Dr Michael Merson, Director of WHO's Global Programme on AIDS. The symposium offered an important opportunity to discuss how best to develop consistent programmes across Europe despite recent political and economic upheavals.

During 1992, the UK continued to contribute towards the costs of WHO's Global Programme on AIDS, and shared UK expertise in a wide variety of meetings and secondments. In addition, bilateral support for 17 national AIDS Control Programmes in Africa, Asia and the Caribbean has been provided, the funds being channelled through the Global Programme. In the EC, projects continued to be supported under the 'Europe against AIDS' programme, the AIDS component of the Biomedicine and Health Research Programme and the AIDS assistance programme for developing countries.

(xiii) Pharmaceuticals

In June, the Council of Ministers formally adopted the Regulation on extended patent protection for pharmaceuticals. This should contribute to the creation of a level playing field for the Japanese, United States and EC pharmaceutical industries.

Among the outstanding Single Market issues resolved during the UK Presidency was the package on Future Systems. This was negotiated by the Medicines Control Agency and is described on page 185.

(xiv) Medical devices

A series of three EC Directives will lead to extensive changes in the control of the safety and marketing of medical devices throughout the Community.

The first, which covers powered implants such as heart pacemakers, comes into effect on 1 January 1993. This Directive provides for a two-year transition period, but from 1 January 1995 all active implantable devices placed on the market or put into service anywhere in the Community must bear a CE marking.

Negotiations on the second Directive, which covers most other devices, continued through 1992. Under the UK Presidency, political agreement at Ministerial level was secured at the Internal Market Council on 17 and 18 December 1992. The provisions of this Directive will come into force on 1 January 1995.

In August 1992, the Commission produced a draft proposal for the third Directive, covering in-vitro diagnostic medical devices. It is expected that a text for further negotiation will be produced early in 1993.

(xv) Research and information technology

The Department continues to be involved in EC health-related research as part of the Third Framework Programme (1990-94). The most important of these for DH is the Biomedical and Health Research Programme (BIOMED 1). It covers four main areas: prevention, care and health systems; major health problems and diseases; the human genome; and biomedical ethics. The other main health-related research initiatives are the Radiation Protection Research Programme - which seeks to improve knowledge about the results of human exposure to radiation - and the Advanced Informatics in Medicine Programme, which seeks to support a common European approach to health care information and telecommunications.

(xvi) Nutrition

Comments were sought on draft regulations to implement the Nutrition Labelling Directive in the UK, and discussions were started about ways to develop nutritional information on food labels to make it easier for consumers to choose healthy diets. The 1991 Committee on Medical Aspects of Food Policy Report on Dietary Reference Values[3] continued to influence the Community, and was especially helpful in the EC Scientific Committee for Food's considerations of the labelling requirements for the Recommended Daily Amounts of vitamins and minerals.

(xvii)   Food safety

Food safety and the Single Market

By the end of 1992, considerable progress had been made towards completion of the Single Market for food. The Community's food law harmonisation programme continued to set high standards of food safety. The Council of Ministers agreed common positions on contaminants in September and on the draft Directive on the Hygiene of Foodstuffs in December. This Directive sets out the broad essentials of food hygiene for the whole food chain from harvesting or slaughter to retail sale, avoiding unnecessarily detailed or intrusive rules, and will provide a sound basis for trade in food across the EC.

Directive on Scientific Co-operation in the Examination of Questions Relating to Food

A common position was reached on this draft Directive in October. It will allow scientific bodies nominated by Member States to carry out food safety evaluations on behalf of the EC. The UK strongly supports this Directive as a way to increase the scientific resources available to the Community.

References

1. *Data Protection Act 1984.* London: HMSO, 1984.
2. *Access to Health Records Act 1990.* London: HMSO, 1990.
3. Department of Health. *Dietary Reference Values for Food Energy and Nutrients for the United Kingdom.* London: HMSO, 1991 (Reports on Health and Social Subjects no. 41).

(c)   Relations with Central and Eastern Europe

Assistance to Central and Eastern Europe was given through several channels.

One of these, the EC's PHARE programme (Poland and Hungary Assistance for Economic Restructuring), supports economic restructuring in Bulgaria, the Czech Republic, Slovakia, Yugoslavia and Romania, as well as Poland and Hungary. PHARE's budget for 1992 was 1,000 million ECU (approximately £800 million), given as non-reimbursable grants to help progress towards a market economy in key areas, including health. There are three main health programmes for Bulgaria, Poland and Romania, and technical assistance programmes are in place for Albania, the Czech Republic, Lithuania and Slovakia.

The UK has bilateral Health Co-operation Agreements with various countries. These facilitated short exchange visits with the former Soviet Union, Poland, Hungary, the Czech Republic, Slovakia, Bulgaria and Romania. British health-care expertise was able to help Europe's emerging democracies in a number of ways. For example, DH organised training in the UK to help doctors from Russia, Belarus and the Ukraine cope with the aftermath of the Chernobyl nuclear accident.

These initiatives were not confined to the public sector. The British Healthcare Consortium (a group of leading health care and pharmaceutical companies) signed an agreement with the Sverdlovsk regional government in the Urals area of Russia to supply health care goods and services. These include hospital design and building, medical equipment supplies, pharmaceuticals, and a programme of health management training put together by NHS Overseas Enterprises (NHSOE) and Manchester University's Health Services Management Unit (HSMU). Officials from NHSOE and HSMU recently visited Yekaterinburg and selected 14 senior managers for the first training programme, which will begin there in the Spring of 1993.

(d)   Council of Europe

DH officials served on the Steering Committee on Bioethics (see page 188) and the European Health Committee. The European Health Committee passed Recommendations on health manpower planning, medico-social aspects of child abuse and standards/guidelines for clinical trials with blood products for consideration for adoption by the Committee of Ministers. It also recommended adoption of a revised technical Protocol to the Agreement on the Exchange of Therapeutic Substances of Human Origin. Expert groups covered the subjects of communication of health information in hospitals, early intervention against HIV infection, the education and training of nurses, and multidisciplinary approaches in the training of health care staff. The UK was represented on all but the last of these groups.

The Department continued to be involved in a number of activities under the Partial Agreement in the health field, notably those that relate to rehabilitation of disabled people and harmonisation of standards and production of guidelines for the use of pesticides, colourings and food additives, detergents, cosmetics and medicines. During the year the UK acted as host for study visits by 65 Fellowship holders from other member countries under the Council of Europe's Fellowship Scheme.

The UK was represented on the European Pharmacopoeia Commission which helped to establish proposals to streamline the future operations of the European Pharmacopoeia; as a result, greater involvement of national Pharmacopoeias and adoption of national monographs should lead to more rapid production of new monographs. During the course of the year the EC acceded to the Pharmacopoeia. The UK promoted the collaborative efforts of the EC and the Council of Europe in their joint programme of biological standardisation. 1992 also saw the move of the European Pharmacopoeia laboratory and the Pharmacopoeia's technical staff to new premises in Strasbourg.

(e) The Commonwealth

The Minister of Health attended the 10th Commonwealth Health Ministers' Conference in Cyprus in October, supported by officials from the Departments of Health and of the Environment. The Conference discussed the serious effects of environmental degradation on the health of communities, individuals and the unborn. It was the first international gathering of Ministers to consider environmental issues after the Earth Summit in Rio (see page 171). Discussion covered health aspects of social and physical environments, waste disposal and sanitation, and food and water safety.

Various projects were proposed to tackle key areas, calling for action on the part of individual Governments, regions and the Commonwealth Secretariat. Proposals to address problems in the social and physical environment involve environmental health training, the establishment of a Commonwealth information network, assistance to develop national strategies, the setting up of pilot schemes to assess environmental health impact and a study to improve the role and status of women.

One Commonwealth-wide and three regional projects were proposed in response to other environmental problems. African members will see proposals for sustainable urban sanitation. The Commonwealth Secretariat will assist in the development of proposals to assess environmental health impact for the Asia-Pacific region, while practical training in solid waste management based on a successful Barbados landfill and water protection model will be made available in the Caribbean. Institutional training links will be set up across the Commonwealth to strengthen the building of environmental health infrastructures in many areas.

A reciprocal health agreement between the UK and Barbados came into force on 1 April 1992.

(f) WHO

(i) European Regional Committee

The 42nd session of the European Regional Committee was held in Copenhagen in September 1992. The UK delegation was led by the Chief Medical Officer. The Regional Director presented his report of WHO's work in Europe during

1991. He drew particular attention to the work carried out under the EUROHEALTH programme of support to the countries of Central and Eastern Europe.

The Regional Committee was mainly occupied with consideration of the proposed programme budget for 1994/95, which was approved. The Regional Director emphasised the severe pressures on the Region's budget arising from the increasing demands of the EUROHEALTH programme. However, the Committee did not sanction a supplementary budget which had sought a 3.5% increase in countries' regular contributions, although it did pass a Resolution urging Member States to make voluntary contributions to the EUROHEALTH programme.

Resolutions were passed in support of an Action Plan for a Tobacco-Free Europe, a European Alcohol Action Plan, and a call for humanitarian assistance to the former Yugoslav republics. A Resolution was also passed to give effect to the proposals of a Committee, chaired by the Chief Medical Officer, which had been set up to consider WHO's European Regional organisation in the light of political changes in Europe. An Interim Standing Committee has been set up to maintain the momentum for change.

(ii) Executive Board

The Executive Board held its 89th Session in Geneva in January 1992. The UK was not entitled to nominate a representative to the Board on this occasion but a member of DH's staff attended as an observer. In his opening statement, the Director General concentrated on the second evaluation of the implementation of the global strategy of 'Health for All by the Year 2000'. He commented on how this had revealed continuing gaps, which in some cases were widening, between rich and poor nations. Members called on WHO to increase its support for primary health care in developing countries. Many argued that development aid often reflected the policies of donors and did not always match the priorities of recipient countries, and that imposition of such policies might adversely affect the ability of poorer countries to develop their own.

The Board approved changes in the programme budget for 1992/93. It was agreed to increase support to programmes covering the organisation of health systems, environmental hazards, immunisation, malaria, diarrhoeal diseases and tuberculosis by making small cuts across other programmes. The Board also considered reports by the Director General on the role of nursing and midwifery, health promotion, disability prevention and rehabilitation, prevention and control of alcohol and drug abuse, immunisation, cholera, health research and AIDS.

The Board discussed the future policy of WHO and decided to set up a Working Group to look at this question in greater depth. In May 1992, the UK again became eligible to put forward a member to serve on the Board and, at the brief Board meeting which followed the World Health Assembly, the Chief Medical Officer was asked to chair this particular Working Group.

(iii) World Health Assembly

The UK Delegation to the 45th World Health Assembly, held in Geneva in May 1992, was led by the Secretary of State for Health. The delegation included representatives from the Overseas Development Administration, which provides funds for many of WHO's special programmes.

In her address to the Assembly, the Secretary of State, referring to the global strategy of 'Health for All by the Year 2000', spoke of the problems facing developing countries and outlined the UK's efforts to alleviate some of these. She told delegates about England's health strategy for the year 2000 and beyond, as set out in the White Paper *The Health of the Nation: a strategy for health in England*[1], and acknowledged a debt to WHO's global strategy. She also spoke of the changes in the UK arising from the Patient's Charter[2] and the reforms of the NHS.

The Assembly discussed the outcome of the second evaluation of the strategy of 'Health for All by the Year 2000'. Member States expressed concern at the widening gap between developed and developing countries - a concern heightened by the belief that recession in the world economy was likely to make matters worse. The Assembly passed a Resolution requesting the Director General to increase further the support given to countries in greatest need, and to give emphasis to the strengthening of health infrastructures and the development of nations' abilities to make efficient use of domestic and external resources to meet health needs.

The Assembly considered reports by the Director General on a range of topics: the role of nursing and midwifery, health promotion, disability prevention and rehabilitation, alcohol and drug abuse, immunisation, health research, technical co-operation, drug policies, health and the environment, child health and development, and AIDS.

Dame Anne Poole, the then Chief Nursing Officer, stressed the need for WHO to strengthen the role of nursing and midwifery. She proposed a Resolution asking the Director General to set up a Global Advisory Group on Nursing and to ensure that the interests of nursing and midwifery were taken into account in policy implementation and programme development.

Technical discussions on the topic of 'Women, Health and Development' covered factors that affected women's health status, morbidity and mortality patterns for women of all ages, and world-wide health-care needs of women, including information, counselling, access to services and legislative support for essential care services. Delegates stressed the particular disadvantages facing women, especially in developing countries.

As well as professional and technological matters, the Assembly also discussed a number of financial and administrative issues. Thirty five Resolutions were passed including those admitting Georgia and Slovenia to full membership of

WHO, and Puerto Rico to associate membership. During the Assembly, Professor David Morley received the Leon Bernard Foundation Prize for his outstanding services in the field of social medicine.

Reference

1. Department of Health. *The Health of the Nation: a strategy for health in England.* London: HMSO, 1992 (Cm. 1986).
2. Department of Health. *The Patient's Charter.* London: Department of Health, 1991.

APPENDIX

Table A.1: *Population age and sex structure, England, 1992, and changes by age, 1981-91 and 1991-92*

Age (in years)	Resident population at mid-1992 (thousands)			Percentage changes (persons)	
	Persons	Males	Females	1981-91	1991-92
Under 1	659	337	322	10.9	-0.6
1-4	2603	1336	1268	15.1	1.2
5-15	6547	3365	3181	-13.2	1.2
16-29	10039	5116	4923	3.8	-1.9
30-44	10147	5082	5064	10.9	-0.2
45-64/59*	9355	5251	4104	0.0	2.8
65/60-74**	5490	1923	3567	-3.0	0.3
75-84	2595	965	1630	16.5	-1.0
85+	792	207	586	49.7	3.5
All ages	48226	23583	24643	2.7	0.3

* 45-64 years for males and 45-59 years for females.

** 65-74 years for males and 60-74 years for females.

Notes: i. The figures for 1992 are projections forward from 1991 estimates provisionally rebased using 1991 Census results. Final rebased 1991 estimates, estimates for mid-1992, and revised historic estimates for the years 1982-90 consistent with these, will all be prepared by OPCS during 1993.

ii. Figures may not add precisely to totals due to rounding.

Source: OPCS

211

Table A.2: *Five main causes of death at different ages (and percentages[1] of all causes of deaths), England, 1992*

RANK	All ages - 1 and over		1-14 years		15-34 years		35-54 years		55-74 years		75 years and over	
	Males	Females	Males	Females	Males	Females	Males	Females	Males	Females	Males	Females
1	Ischaemic heart disease	Ischaemic heart disease	Road vehicle accidents	Congenital anomalies	Road vehicle accidents	Road vehicle accidents	Ischaemic heart disease	MN* of bone, connective tissue, skin and breast	Ischaemic heart disease	Ischaemic heart disease	Ischaemic heart disease	Ischaemic heart disease
	29%	23%	18%	15%	21%	14%	28%	22%	34%	24%	27%	25%
2	Cerebro-vascular disease	Cerebro-vascular disease	Other causes of injury and poisoning†	Other causes of injury and poisoning†	Other causes of injury and poisoning†	Other causes of injury and poisoning†	MN* of digestive organs and peritoneum	MN* of genito-urinary organs	MN* of respiratory and intra-thoracic organs	MN* of digestive organs and peritoneum	Cerebro-vascular disease	Cerebro-vascular disease
	9%	15%	16%	15%	20%	12%	9%	10%	13%	10%	12%	17%
3	MN* of respiratory and intra-thoracic organs	MN* of digestive organs and peritoneum	Congenital anomalies	Diseases of the nervous system and sense organs	Suicide and self-inflicted injury	Suicide and self-inflicted injury	MN* of respiratory and intra-thoracic organs	MN* of digestive organs and peritoneum	MN* of digestive organs and peritoneum	Cerebro-vascular disease	Chronic obstructive pulmonary disease and allied conditions	Pneumonia
	9%	7%	11%	13%	17%	9%	8%	9%	10%	9%	8%	8%
4	MN* of digestive organs and peritoneum	Pneumonia	Diseases of the nervous system and sense organs	Road vehicle accidents	Diseases of the nervous system and sense organs	Diseases of the nervous system and sense organs	Other causes of injury and poisoning†	Ischaemic heart disease	Cerebro-vascular disease	MN* of respiratory and intra-thoracic organs	MN* of respiratory and intra-thoracic organs	MN* of digestive organs and peritoneum
	8%	6%	11%	11%	5%	8%	6%	8%	7%	8%	7%	6%
5	Chronic obstructive pulmonary disease and allied conditions	MN* of bone, connective tissue, skin and breast	MN* of lymphatic and haematopoietic tissue	MN* of lymphatic and haematopoietic tissue	MN* of lymphatic and haematopoietic tissue	MN* of bone, connective tissue, skin and breast	Suicide and self-inflicted injury	MN* of respiratory and intra-thoracic organs	Chronic obstructive pulmonary disease and allied conditions	MN* of bone, connective tissue, skin and breast	MN* of digestive organs and peritoneum	Mental disorders
	7%	5%	7%	5%	4%	7%	6%	7%	6%	8%	7%	4%
Remainder	38%	44%	36%	41%	33%	51%	43%	45%	30%	41%	39%	40%
All causes of death	251751	266646	996	726	5864	2579	17788	11243	102354	88888	124749	183210

[1] May not add up to 100 due to rounding. * MN = malignant neoplasm.

† 'Other causes of injury and poisoning' comprises categories of external injury and poisoning (E800-E999) excluding road vehicle accidents (E810-E829) and suicide (E950-E959).

Source: OPCS

Table A.3: Relative mortality from various conditions when presented as numbers of deaths and future years of 'working life' lost, England and Wales, 1992

Cause (ICD9 code)	Males				Females			
	Number of deaths (thousands)		Years of 'working life' lost (thousands)		Number of deaths (thousands)		Years of 'working life' lost (thousands)	
	All ages	(%)	Age 15-64	(%)	All ages	(%)	Age 15-64	(%)
All causes, all ages	272		915		287		544	
All causes, 28 days and over	270	(100)	832	(100)	285	(100)	480	(100)
All malignant neoplasms* (140-208)	75	(28)	183	(22)	64	(22)	195	(41)
Lung cancer (162)	23	(9)	39	(5)	10	(4)	20	(4)
Breast cancer+ (174)					13	(5)	59	(12)
Genito-urinary cancer (179-189)	14	(5)	16	(2)	9	(3)	35	(7)
Leukaemia (204-208)	2	(1)	14	(2)	2	(1)	16	(3)
Circulatory disease* (390-459)	122	(45)	201	(24)	124	(44)	74	(15)
Ischaemic heart disease (410-414)	79	(29)	144	(17)	67	(24)	32	(7)
Cerebrovascular disease (430-438)	25	(9)	26	(3)	39	(14)	23	(5)
Respiratory disease* (460-519)	30	(11)	36	(4)	31	(11)	21	(4)
Pneumonia (480-486)	9	(3)	14	(2)	16	(6)	6	(1)
Bronchitis, emphysema and asthma (490-493)	5	(2)	9	(1)	3	(1)	7	(1)
Sudden infant death syndrome (798.0)	0	(0)	15	(2)	0	(0)	8	(2)
All accidental deaths* (E800-E949)	6	(2)	131	(16)	4	(1)	39	(8)
Motor vehicle traffic accidents (E810-E819)	3	(1)	77	(9)	1	(0)	23	(5)
Suicide (E950-E959)	3	(1)	67	(8)	1	(0)	15	(3)

* These conditions are ranked as well as selected causes within these broader headings.   + Not calculated for male breast cancer.

Deaths under 28 days are excluded, except from 'All causes, all ages'.

Source: OPCS

Table A.4: *Trends in 'avoidable' deaths, England and Wales, 1979-92. Age-standardised mortality ratios (1979 = 100)*

Condition	SMR[1]												Actual number of deaths[4]	
	1979	1982	1983	1984	1985	1986	1987	1988	1989	1990	1991	1992	1979	1992
Hypertension/cerebrovascular (ages 35-64)	100	84	80	77	76	72	68	63	60	57	57*	55	9482	5181
Perinatal mortality[2]	100	77	71	69	67	65	61	60	57	55	55	51	9400	5213
Cervical cancer (ages 15-64)	100	90	90	91	91	97	89	84	80	77	73	68	1142	785
Hodgkin's disease (ages 5-64)	100	86	86	79	75	74	82	74	64	59	57*	59	365	229
Respiratory diseases (ages 1-14)	100	87	62	51	50	40	47	40	41	39	41	28	329	93
Surgical diseases[3] (ages 5-64)	100	77	71	78	66	72	53	69	52	58	55	60	262	155
Asthma (ages 5-44)	100	105	105	102	113	111	111	106	92	84	88	68	250	183
Tuberculosis (ages 5-64)	100	91	62	64	65	58	63	55	55	47	47	47	222	106
Chronic rheumatic heart disease (ages 5-44)	100	52	42	41	35	34	32	18	26	21	19	14	133	22
Total 'avoidable' deaths	100	81	76	74	72	70	66	62	59	57	57	54	21585	11967
All causes: ages 0-14 years	100	82	77	73	74	73	72	71	66	62	58	54	11132	6450
All causes: ages 15-64 years	100	92	90	88	88	86	84	82	80	78	76	74	127194	94491
All causes: all ages	100	94	93	89	92	89	86	85	85	82	82	84	591039	558313

[1] The standardised mortality ratio (SMR) for a condition is calculated by dividing the observed number of deaths by the expected number of deaths based on 1979 death rates.

[2] Stillbirths (2,929 in 1992) are included in perinatal mortality and total 'avoidable' deaths, but not in deaths from all causes.

[3] Appendicitis, abdominal hernia, cholelithiasis and cholecystitis.

[4] Excluding deaths of visitors to England and Wales.

* Revised from figure (58) quoted in 1991 Report.

Source: Calculated by Department of Health (SD2A) from data supplied by OPCS

Table A.5: Live births, stillbirths, infant mortality and abortions, England[1], 1960-92

Year	Live births Number	Stillbirths Number	Stillbirths Rate[2]	Early neonatal mortality (deaths under 1 week) Number	Early neonatal mortality (deaths under 1 week) Rate[3]	Perinatal mortality (stillbirths plus deaths under 1 week) Rate[2]	Post-neonatal mortality (deaths 4 weeks to under 1 year) Rate[3]	Infant mortality (deaths under 1 year) Rate[3]	Abortions[1] Rate[4]
1960	740859	14753	19.5	9772	13.2	32.5	6.3	21.6	-
1970	741999	9708	12.9	7864	10.6	23.4	5.9	18.2	87.6
1975	563900	5918	10.4	5154	9.1	19.4	5.0	15.7	149.9
1976	550393	5339	9.6	4468	8.1	17.6	4.6	14.2	148.7
1977	536953	5087	9.4	4070	7.6	16.9	4.5	13.7	152.7
1978	562589	4791	8.4	3975	7.1	15.4	4.4	13.1	157.7
1979	601316	4811	7.9	4028	6.7	14.6	4.5	12.8	158.8
1980	619371	4523	7.3	3793	6.1	13.4	4.4	12.0	164.5
1981	598163	3939	6.5	3105	5.2	11.7	4.3	10.9	168.8
1982	589711	3731	6.3	2939	5.0	11.2	4.5*	10.8	171.1
1983	593255	3412	5.7	2746	4.6	10.3	4.2	10.0	169.2
1984	600573	3425	5.7	2640	4.4	10.0	3.9	9.4	177.3
1985	619301	3426	5.5	2674	4.3	9.8	3.9	9.2	177.6
1986	623609	3337	5.3	2640	4.2	9.5	4.2	9.5	183.5
1987	643330	3224	5.0	2518	3.9	8.9	4.0	9.1	187.7
1988	654360	3188	4.8	2543	3.9	8.7	4.1	9.1	196.6
1989	649357	3056	4.7	2368	3.6	8.3	3.7	8.4	200.0
1990	666920	3068	4.6	2382	3.6	8.1	3.3	7.9	199.0
1991	660806	3072	4.6	2260	3.4	8.0	3.0	7.3	194.4
1992	651784	2777††	4.2†	2174	3.3	7.6†	2.3	6.5	190.1[5]

[1] Relates to England residents. [2] Per 1,000 live and stillbirths. [3] Per 1,000 live births. [4] Per 1,000 conceptions (live births, stillbirths and abortions). [5] Provisional.

* The post-neonatal mortality rate in 1982 has been incorrectly cited as 4.6 per 1,000 live births in recent Reports.

†† 1992 figures exclude 198 stillbirths of between 24 and 27 completed weeks gestation registered between 1 October 1992 and 31 December 1992, following the introduction of new legislation (see Chapter 1).

Source: OPCS

Table A.6: Congenital malformations, England, 1980, 1985, 1991† and 1992†

ICD Code(s)	Malformation	Live births*				Stillbirths**			
		1980	1985	1991	1992#	1980	1985	1991	1992#
	Malformed babies								
	Number	12704	12215	6482	5618	619	322	186	175
	Rate	205.4	197.2	98.1	86.2	9.9	5.2	2.8	2.7
320-359, 740, 741, 742.0-742.5, 742.8, 742.9, 767.6	Central nervous system								
	Number	1087	679	288	272	626	148	43	52
	Rate	17.6	11.0	4.4	4.2	10.0	2.4	0.6	0.8
360-389, 743.0-743.6, 743.8-744.3	Ear and eye								
	Number	446	686	327	232	22	21	10	8
	Rate	7.2	11.1	4.9	3.6	0.4	0.3	0.2	0.1
749.0-749.2	Cleft lip/cleft palate								
	Number	815	758	716	678	49	19	13	12
	Rate	13.2	12.2	10.8	10.4	0.8	0.3	0.2	0.2
390-459, 745-747, 785.2	Cardiovascular								
	Number	817	794	531	504	16	12	16	7
	Rate	13.2	12.8	8.0	7.7	0.3	0.2	0.2	0.1
752.6	Hypospadias/epispadias								
	Number	930	1001	691	521	1	3	2	1
	Rate	15.0	16.2	10.5	8.0	0.0	0.0	0.0	0.0
755.0, 755.1	Polydactyly/syndactyly								
	Number	986	1097	879	741	21	18	6	11
	Rate	15.9	17.7	13.3	11.4	0.3	0.3	0.1	0.2
754.5-754.7	Talipes								
	Number	2318	1873	859	738	43	19	5	4
	Rate	37.5	30.2	13.0	11.3	0.7	0.3	0.1	0.1
758.0-758.9	Chromosomal								
	Number	523	520	502	468	16	16	23	16
	Rate	8.5	8.4	7.6	7.2	0.3	0.3	0.3	0.2

† From January 1990 certain minor malformations are no longer notified, and have been excluded from the figures shown. For example, club foot of positional origin is now excluded from the category 'Talipes', ICD Codes 754.5-754.7. This change in notification practice largely accounts for the decrease in the number of malformations reported in some categories.

* Rates per 10,000 live births.   ** Rates per 10,000 total births.   # Provisional data.

Source: OPCS

Table A.7: Cancer* registrations by sex, age and site: males, England and Wales, 1988

Numbers and percentages

Age-group (years)

	All ages	%	0-14 years	%	15-24 years	%	25-44 years	%	45-64 years	%	65-74 years	%	75-84 years	%	85 and over	%
Eye, brain and other nervous system	2095	2	156	22	101	11	343	7	823	3	463	1	192	1	17	0
Mouth and pharynx	2114	2	4	1	19	2	160	3	867	3	587	1	395	1	82	1
Oesophagus	3044	3	1	0	1	0	75	1	907	3	1108	3	769	2	183	3
Lung	26542	22	3	0	3	0	318	6	7212	22	10269	25	7445	22	1292	18
Stomach	6942	6	2	0	4	0	125	2	1702	5	2457	6	2234	7	418	6
Pancreas	3066	3	2	0	4	0	79	2	857	3	1052	3	875	3	197	3
Large intestine and rectum	13456	11	6	1	14	2	368	7	3640	11	4586	11	3980	12	862	12
Prostate	12496	10	2	0	2	0	11	0	1540	5	4453	11	5202	15	1286	18
Bladder	8265	7	8	1	8	1	162	3	2219	7	2885	7	2433	7	550	8
Skin (melanoma)†	1494	1	10	1	44	5	402	8	548	2	279	1	179	1	32	0
Leukaemias and lymphomas	8248	7	303	43	319	35	849	16	2315	7	2249	6	1766	5	447	6
All other cancer	32772	27	203	29	391	43	2306	44	9447	29	10413	26	8129	24	1883	26
Total cancer	120534	100	700	100	910	100	5198	100	32077	100	40801	100	33599	100	7249	100

* Cancer = malignant neoplasm.

† Melanoma of skin only (ICD9 code 172). Earlier reports included figures for other malignant neoplasm of skin (ICD9 code 173), which are greatly under-registered.

Note: i. The bulk of the apparent increase of just over 10% in the figures for registrations in 1988 compared with those published for 1987 is artefactual. A problem with the transmission of data from one registry was resolved; revised figures for 1987 and some earlier years will be given in the OPCS Annual Reference Volume for 1988.

ii. Percentages may not add up to 100 due to rounding.

Source: OPCS

217

Table A.8: Cancer* registrations by sex, age and site: females, England and Wales, 1988

Numbers and percentages

Age-group (years)

	All ages	%	0-14 years	%	15-24 years	%	25-44 years	%	45-64 years	%	65-74 years	%	75-84 years	%	85 and over	%
Eye, brain and other nervous system	1673	1	124	22	69	9	262	3	579	2	405	1	201	1	33	0
Mouth and pharynx	1180	1	10	2	13	2	76	1	346	1	353	1	280	1	102	1
Oesophagus	2129	2	1	0	0	0	34	0	388	1	567	2	806	3	333	3
Breast	26702	22	4	1	27	3	3291	35	10376	31	6188	19	4855	15	1964	16
Lung	11774	10	1	0	2	0	221	2	3343	10	4353	14	3075	10	776	6
Stomach	4305	4	1	0	2	0	76	1	599	2	1082	3	1738	6	807	7
Pancreas	3171	3	1	0	4	1	40	0	577	2	924	3	1141	4	484	4
Large intestine and rectum	13889	12	6	1	11	1	347	4	2816	8	3842	12	4799	15	2068	17
Ovary	5174	4	15	3	50	6	445	5	2050	6	1376	4	950	3	288	2
Cervix	4467	4	2	0	53	7	1576	17	1476	4	804	3	429	1	127	1
Other uterus	4197	3	1	0	3	0	162	2	1706	5	1235	4	818	3	272	2
Bladder	3305	3	4	1	4	1	72	1	710	2	967	3	1134	4	414	3
Skin (melanoma)†	2388	2	9	2	100	13	631	7	793	2	450	1	293	1	112	1
Leukaemias and lymphomas	7227	6	206	36	248	32	631	7	1590	5	1737	5	2061	7	754	6
All other cancer	28455	24	184	32	195	25	1480	16	6352	19	7653	24	8858	28	3733	30
Total cancer	120036	100	569	100	781	100	9344	100	33701	100	31936	100	31438	100	12267	100

* Cancer = malignant neoplasm.

† Melanoma of skin only (ICD9 code 172). Earlier reports included figures for other malignant neoplasm of skin (ICD9 code 173).

Note: i. The bulk of the apparent increase of just over 10% in the figures for registrations in 1988 compared with those published for 1987 is artefactual. A problem with the transmission of data from one registry was resolved; revised figures for 1987 and some earlier years will be given in the OPCS Annual Reference Volume for 1988.

ii. Percentages may not add up to 100 due to rounding.

Source: OPCS

218

Table A9: *Percentage of children immunised by their 2nd birthday and of children given BCG vaccine by their 14th birthday, England, 1980-91/92*

Year	Diphtheria	Tetanus	Polio	Whooping cough	Measles	Mumps/ Rubella	BCG[1]
1980[2]	81	81	81	41	53	-	82
1981[2]	83	83	82	46	55	-	78
1982[2]	84	84	84	53	58	-	75
1983[2]	84	84	84	59	60	-	76
1984[2]	84	84	84	65	63	-	71
1985[2]	85	85	85	65	68	-	77
1986[2]	85	85	85	67	71	-	76
1987/88[2]	87	87	87	73	76	-	76
1988/89	87	87	87	75	80	7	71
1989/90	89	89	89	78	84	68	36[3]
1990/91	92	92	92	84	87	86	90
1991/92	93	93	93	88	90	90	86

1 Estimated percentage.
2 Estimated percentage immunised by the end of the second year after birth.
3 The school BCG programme was suspended in 1989 because there were insufficient supplies of BCG vaccine.

Sources: 1980-87/88: Form SBL 607
1988/89 onwards: Form KC51 (except BCG); KC50 (BCG)

Table A.10: *Cumulative totals of AIDS cases by exposure category, England, to 31 December 1992*

(Numbers subject to revision as further data are received or duplicates identified)

How persons probably acquired the virus	Number of cases			
	Male	Female	Total	%+
Sexual intercourse:				
between men	5003	0	5003	78
between men and women				
'High risk' partner*	21	41	62	1
Other partner abroad**	298	184	482	7
Other partner UK	28	23	51	1
Not known	4	0	4	<1
Injecting drug use (IDU)	143	59	202	3
IDU and sexual intercourse				
between men	105	0	105	2
Blood				
Blood factor (eg haemophiliacs)	294	5	299	5
Blood or tissue transfer (eg transfusion)				
Abroad	13	30	43	1
UK	14	15	29	1
Mother to child	34	35	69	1
Other/undetermined	72	12	84	1
Total	6029	404	6433	100

* Includes men and women who had sex with injecting drug users, or with those infected through blood factor treatment or blood transfusion, and women who had sex with bisexual men.

** Includes persons without other identified risks who are from, or who have lived in, countries where the major route of HIV-1 transmission is through sexual intercourse between men and women.

+ Total does not add up to 100 because of rounding.

Source: CDSC

Figure A1: *Weekly deaths, England and Wales, 1991 and 1992, and expected deaths 1992*

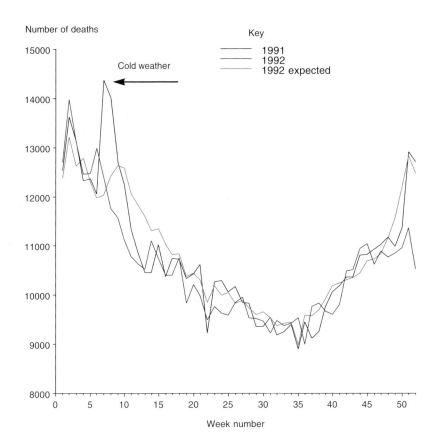

Notes: i.   The following weeks have been averaged to take account of the Easter and Christmas holidays: week 52 1990 and week 1 1991; weeks 13 and 14 1991; week 52 1991 and week 1 1992; weeks 16 and 17 1992; and week 52 1992 and week 1 1993.
  ii. Data are for 1-year-olds and over.

Source: OPCS